Neurosurgery Lecture Notes

An International Curriculum

Neurosurgery Lecture Notes

An International Curriculum

W. Adriaan Liebenberg
MMed Neurosurgery (Stellenbosch), FCS Neurosurg (SA)

Lal Gunasekera
Phd, FRCS

With contributions from

Andreas K. Demetriades
B.Sc (Honours), M.Phil (Cantab)
MRCS (Ed & Eng)

VESUVIUS BOOKS LTD
Published by Vesuvius Books Ltd.
Copyright © Vesuvius Books Ltd, 2006

All rights reserved. No part of this publication may be translated into other languages, reproduced, stored in a retrieval system, or transmitted, in any form or by any means, electronic, mechanical, photocopying, recording or otherwise, without prior permission in writing of the publisher.

No responsibility or liability is assumed by either the authors or the publisher for any injury, loss, or damage to persons or property as a matter of products liability, negligence, or otherwise, or from the use or operation of any methods, products, instruments, instructions, or ideas contained in this book. Every effort has been made to ensure that the details given in this book regarding the choice, operation or use of any instrumentation, or the choice, dosage and administration practices relating to pharmaceutical agents, which are mentioned in the text, are in accordance with the recommendations and practices current at the time of publication. However, because new research constantly leads to such recommendations and practices being updated, the reader should obtain independent verification of diagnoses and check the makers' instructions carefully regarding the choice and use of instruments, and regarding the administration practices, doses, indications and contraindications associated with pharmaceutical agents mentioned in this book.

The statements made, and the opinions expressed, in this book are those of the authors and do not necessarily reflect the views of the company or companies which manufacture and/or market any of the instruments or pharmaceutical products referred to, nor do any statement made amounts to an endorsement of the quality or value of such instruments or products, or any claims made by their manufacturers.

ISBN 0-9548813-1-1

This book is dedicated to the memory of Ryno Conradie

He was a prince of a man, a loving husband and a doting father. May he rest in peace.

Jy sal nie vergeet word nie.

Contents

1. Modern neurosurgery
2. Clinical evaluation
3. Cranial imaging
4. Spinal imaging
5. Cranial and spinal tumours
6. Vascular abnormalities
7. Cerebral infarction and haemorrhage
8. Raised intracranial pressure
9. Craniospinal injury
10. Diseases of the spine
11. Nerve entrapment and disorders of peripheral nerves
12. Congenital abnormalities
13. Infection
14. ICU management
15. Theatre
16. Further reading

Introduction

I fell into neurosurgery completely by chance but became hooked on it as soon as I arrived in the department. I have never looked back and have come to have a love-hate relationship with this tough taskmaster that is neurosurgery.

It is a specialty where you can truly make a difference in people's lives but at the same time it is a specialty where some conditions have a hopeless prognosis and this demands a very special approach. It is a road less traveled and therefore attracts a certain type of person. These are usually high achievers and driven people who have a certain vision in life.

A neurosurgical attachment can be ardous or it can be a useful and elightening experience. The first time you see the remarkable recovery that patient's with blocked shunts or chronic subdural haematomas have, you cannot help but be awed by the awesome power you wield with simple procedures not far removed from what ancient peoples used to do. You might experience the life changing effect that functional surgery can have in patients lives that suffer intractable pain, epilepsy or movement disorders. The effect that disc surgery has - especially in the cervical region - is also remarkable to see. At the same time it is difficult not to marvel at the enthusiasm and tenacity that neurosurgeons display when attacking incurable brain cancer to be able to afford their patients prolonged quality of life.

There is much more to neurosurgery than meets the eye and my wish is that you have the opportunity of delving into this specialty and be able to snoop around a bit to see what it might offer.

Adriaan Liebenberg

1

MODERN NEUROSURGERY

Contents

Introduction
Skull base neurosurgeons
Spinal neurosurgeons
Vascular neurosurgeons
Pituitary neurosurgeons
Paediatric neurosurgeons
Functional neurosurgeons
Neurosurgeons treating pain
Trauma neurosurgeons
Oncological neurosurgeons
Radiation neurosurgeons
General neurosurgeons

Introduction
The specialty of neurosurgery, like most other specialties in medicine is subdivided into sub-specialties. Neurosurgical units will frequently employ neurosurgeons for their skill and experience in dealing with a particular sub-specialty of neurosurgery. It commonly follows a period where the surgeon worked in that specific sub section of neurosurgery under the supervision of a recognised leader in that area. These are commonly called fellowships. Sub-specialisation is especially prevalent in developed countries where the ratio of neurosurgeon to patient is favourable, whereas the pressures of too few surgeons in the developing countries leads to an approach of generalist neurosurgeons that treat the whole spectrum of neurosurgery. The following are some of the subtypes of neurosurgical specialties:

Skull base neurosurgeons treat conditions in the region of the skull base. This includes tumours and other lesions on the clivus, dorsum sellae, sphenoid ridge, petrous bone, in the cerebellopontine angle, around the third ventricle and foramen magnum. These surgeons need to be excellent anatomists as the approaches are fraught with danger. There are a multitude of very important nerves and blood vessels running through the skull base and as they are encased in bones and passing through foramina, they frequently have to be meticulously drilled out with high speed drills. Degenerative conditions that are treated include rheumatoid arthritis which leads to skull base settling and instability and resultant myelopathy (spasticity or stiffness of the limbs). Decompression and fixation is usually indicated in patients who have progressive symptoms. Herniation of the cerebellum into the upper cervical canal in Arnold Chiari malformation also leads to myelopathy and bulbar symptoms and is treated by decompression.

Spinal neurosurgeons decompress the spinal cord and nerve roots with removal of compressive bony elements and discogenic material via laminectomies, discectomies, foraminotomies and anterior approaches. They may also fuse the vertebral column with instrumentation and bony fusion to treat instability.

Vascular neurosurgeons treat vascular abnormalities in patients who present with haemorrhages or neurological dysfunction secondary to arteriovenous malformations or aneurysms. They do this by excluding the lesions from the circulation or by obliterating them. They also perform bypass operations on blood vessels and endarterectomies, where they remove atherosclerotic plaques obstructing blood flow. Sometimes they use stents to maintain the integrity of blood vessels.

Pituitary neurosurgeons are frequently skull base neurosurgeons or vascular neurosurgeons and treat adenomas arising in the pituitary fossa from the hypophysis. Surgery is employed in cases where medical therapy failed to control hormone producing adenomas and, in cases of non hormone producing adenomas, to prevent blindness where there is compression of the optic nerves. Most pituitary tumours can be removed from below, by approaching through the sphenoidal sinus. However very large tumours can also have a compressive effect on brain tissue and these often have to be removed by combining the traditional approach from below with a craniotomy to approach the lesion from above. Pituitary neurosurgeons frequently have some cross over with skull base surgery or vascular surgery.

Pediatric neurosurgeons treat pathology in children similar to those in adult patients plus the developmental abnormalities seen in the first few years of life.

Functional neurosurgeons treat epilepsy, movement disorders and sometimes psychiatric disorders with stereotactically guided surgery. The actual surgery is frequently minor as far as the size of the insult is concerned but because it is performed in extremely eloquent areas, the positioning and lesioning has to be exceedingly accurate.

Neurosurgeons treating pain manage a variety of syndromes including the neurovascular compression syndromes and intractable dysaesthetic pain. They may use neurovascular decompressions, spinal stimulators, rhizotomies and stimulation/ablation of areas of the brain such as the peri-aquaductal grey area or areas of the thalamus. They frequently have to work together with the spinal surgeons to treat patients who have failed back surgery syndrome (intractable pain and variable degrees of functional incapacitation following back surgery)

Trauma neurosurgeons, trauma is usually managed by the general neurosurgeon. However some surgeons specialise in this field and might incorporate Intensive Care Unit training into their education. The pathology seen includes cranial soft tissue damage, skull fracture, traumatic haemorrhage and a variety of spinal trauma.

Oncological neurosurgeons deal with resection of tumours and biopsy for diagnostic purposes to facilitate adjunctive therapies like radiotherapy or chemotherapy. Even though brain tumours are fairly scarce in the general population, this is a very busy sub speciality and can be emotionally draining, especially pediatric oncology.

Types of neurosurgeons	What do they do?
Skull base neurosurgeons	Treat conditions of the skull base (clivus, dorsum sellae, sphenoid ridge, petrous bone, in the cerebellopontine angle, around the third ventricle and Foramen Magnum.)
Spinal neurosurgeons	Decompress neural structures in the spinal canal and stabilise the spine with fusions.
Vascular neurosurgeons	Treat vascular abnormalities by excision or occlusion of these abnormalities. They also perform bypass operations, endarterectomies or place stents in critically stenosed vessels.
Pituitary neurosurgeons	Treat hypophyseal adenomas in the pituitary fossa surgically when medical therapy fails or is not indicated
Pediatric neurosurgeons	Treat pathology in children similar to those in adult patients plus the developmental abnormalities seen in the first few years of life.
Functional neurosurgeons	Treat epilepsy, movement disorders and sometimes psychiatric disorders with stereotactically guided surgery.
Neurosurgeons treating pain	Treat a variety of syndromes including the neurovascular compression syndromes and intractable dysaesthetic pain.
Trauma neurosurgeons	Treat cranial soft tissue damage, skull fractures, traumatic haemorrhage and a variety of spinal trauma.
Oncological neurosurgeons	Treat tumours with resection and biopsy for diagnostic purposes to facilitate adjunctive therapies like radiotherapy and/or chemotherapy.
Radiation neurosurgeons	Treat patients with focused beam radiotherapy for a variety of pathology including tumours and vascular lesions.
General neurosurgeons	Treat a variety of conditions including trauma, spinal conditions, oncology, CSF diversion, craniocervical junction surgery and peripheral nerve surgery.

Some neurosurgeons treat patients with external radiation. The Linnac particle beam accelerator (conventional radiation beams) and the Gamma knife (Cobalt 60 source) are two external radiation sources that can be focused on a very small area of brain and have a minimal effect on surrounding structures. The practice of using whole brain radiation is used for widespread and aggressive tumours as well as those that have the propensity to metastasise.

General neurosurgeons deal with more than one sub speciality that can include trauma, spinal conditions, oncology, CSF diversion, craniospinal junction surgery and peripheral nerve surgery.

There has to be close co-operation and communication between neurosurgeons that sub-specialise in units to ensure adequate treatment of patients. To make on call commitments more acceptable, there might sometimes be a supraregional service where for instance the vascular neurosurgeons of several centres cross cover for each other.

It is probable that in the first world there will be a continued movement towards sub specialisation as the public demands and scrutiny grows in this delicate surgical field. In the third world the true generalist neurosurgeon will continue on for some time yet.

2

CLINICAL EVALUATION

Contents

Introduction
History
Physical Examination

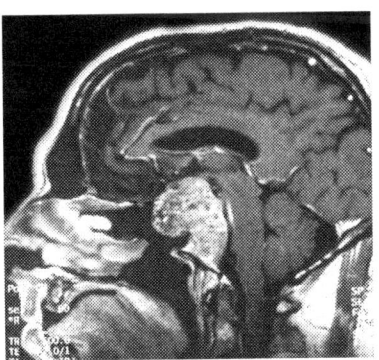

Introduction

Clinical evaluation of a neurosurgical patient as in any other specialty is directed towards arriving at a diagnosis. The diagnosis consists of :

1. Where is the disease? (in terms of anatomy) and
2. What is the disease? (in terms of pathology)

To assist in determining the above you have to take a careful history which will enable you to focus your attention on a particular region of the CNS and conduct a physical examination with emphasis on that particular region. As in other specialties this can involve inspection where the diseased organ can be seen (e.g. the optic fundus), palpation where the organ can be felt (e.g. spinal deformities), and in certain instances auscultation where blood flow changes with disease. These methods have limited direct application to the central nervous system (CNS).

Thus, the diagnosis of a neurological disorder usually requires a different approach. The brain and the spinal cord and even the peripheral nerves are highly specialised structures and in different areas control different functions. Hence if any area in the CNS is diseased, the function controlled by that area will be affected. If you determine what functions are affected in the patient, you can relate these to the area of the CNS involved and thereby determine where the lesion is (in terms of the anatomy). For example, speech is controlled by the speech area situated in the left hemisphere in the temporal region in right handed persons and most left handed persons as well (a proportion of left handed patients have their speech area on the right side). If speech is impaired in a patient, the disease can be localised to the left temporal region of the brain indicating where the lesion is.

The pathology can be determined from the history of onset of the symptoms. The common neurosurgical disorders can be classified as congenital, traumatic, degenerative, inflammatory, neoplastic or vascular diseases. In most congenital disorders the symptoms would be apparent from birth, in traumatic conditions there would be a history of an injury and in inflammatory diseases, there may be features such as pyrexia to suggest infection. As neoplasms grow slowly, the symptoms appear slowly and progress. In vascular diseases blood vessels either get blocked or burst suddenly and the symptoms also are sudden in onset, so much so that the patient or an observer could usually recall exactly what they were doing when it happened. Thus, the history of onset and the progression of symptoms indicate the pathology and the functional impairment determined mainly by the examination points towards the anatomy. Together they help to arrive at the diagnosis.

History

The history is directed mainly towards what functional changes the patient has noticed and the mode of onset and progression. The history should also include a careful past medical history as the present problem may be related to a past illness. The family history is important as many neurological diseases have a hereditary tendency. Drug history and occupational history may indicate exposure to any hazards that could have contributed to the disease. Personal habits such as smoking and alcohol abuse are also relevant in some instances. Social history is important as many neurological diseases can lead to a chronic disability that would have a considerable social impact on the family and friends. Finally a systematic enquiry helps to determine any other co-existing illness which may be relevant to the neurological illness.

Physical Examination

As the diagnosis of neurological diseases involves a careful scrutiny of functional deficits, you have to examine all the functions of the CNS to find out which are impaired. This involves a systematic approach in order not to miss anything and this process constitutes the neurological examination.

The steps involved are:

1. Vital signs
These are pulse rate, blood pressure, respiratory rate and temperature. These signs being measured and expressed in numerical terms are hence objective and any changes can be quantified. They also change with changes of intracranial dynamics and hence form an important aspect in the evaluation and subsequent observation of a neurosurgical patient.

2. Systemic examination
It is preferable for all other systems to be examined first before concentrating on the neurological examination as symptoms of diseases of these systems can mimic neurological diseases (e.g. confusion caused by anoxia). Also, the neurological disturbance could very well be secondary to a systemic illness (e.g. metastatic tumours, cerebral infarcts from cardiac emboli etc.).

3. Neurological examination
(See below)

Neurological examination

The full and thorough examination of a neurosurgical patient should be a seamless, fast process and comes only with practice. Following the detailed history you will already have a very good idea of what it is that you are dealing with and you can tailor your examination to this. When there is a good understanding of the pathology it becomes quite easy to focus on certain aspects.

Alertness and mental function
Patients with neurological disease frequently have differing levels of consciousness and examination of unconscious patients obviously differs markedly from that of the patient who is conscious, awake and alert. In the patient who is awake the first thing to assess is their mental function and orientation in time, place and person. Two bedside tests are the abbreviated mental test score and the mini mental state examination. See tables 1 and 2.

These are quite rough tools which will not pick up subtle deficiencies, so if these are suspected then assessment by a neuropsychologist is indicated. This is especially true in those patients who are recuperating from an insult to the nervous system such as subarachnoid haemorrhage or traumatic brain injury. It is always good to quantify a baseline in these patients so that progression and improvement can be seen. Following the testing of mental function and orientation of the patient it should be recorded as follows: AMT (score)/10 and MMSE (score)/30 with the orientation noted as "orientated in time, place and person."

Cranial nerves
CN I
The first cranial nerve is frequently involved in tumours of the anterior skull base or in trauma of the anterior skull base and can be tested with different substances. Oil of cloves or coffee is frequently used. The olfactory nerves can be tested independently by pinching the opposite nostril shut and testing one side at a time.

CN II
Visual fields. The second cranial nerve carries visual signals from the retina to the occipital cortex. Compression of the optic nerve or the optic tract and its radiations will lead to deficiencies in the visual field. There will be different clinical manifestations depending on where the compression is. See figure 1. Deficiencies are diagnosed with confrontation testing. See figure 2.

Visual acuity. Visual acuity is tested with a Snellen chart over a set distance of 20 feet and noted as a value which is a fraction of one. Therefore, if the set distance is 20 feet and the patient can see the letters that the chart indicates you should be able to see over a distance of 20 foot and therefore has 20/20 vision, it indicates a value of one, which is normal. If the patient can only see the large letters which you should be able to read at 200 feet then the vision is recorded as 20/200 or 1/10 of normal vision. Countries with the metric system use

Task	Instructions	Scoring	
Orientation (Date)	"Tell me the date?" Ask for omitted items	One point each for year, season, date, day of week, and month	5
Orientation (Place)	"Where are you?" Ask for omitted items	One point each for state, county, town, building, and floor or room	5
Register 3 objects	Name three objects slowly and clearly. Ask the patient to repeat them	One point for each item correctly repeated	3
Serial sevens	Ask the patient to count backwards from 100 by 7. Stop after five answers. (Or ask them to spell "world" backwards)	One point for each correct answer (or letter)	5
Recall 3 objects	Ask the patient to recall the objects mentioned above	One point for each item correctly remembered	3
Naming	Point to your watch and ask the patient "what is this?" Repeat with a pencil.	One point for each correct answer	2
Repeating a phrase	Ask the patient to say "no ifs, ands, or buts"	One point if successful on first try	1
Verbal commands	Give the patient a plain piece of paper and say "Take this paper in your right hand, fold it in half, and put it on the floor"	One point for each correct action	3
Written commands	Show the patient a piece of paper with "CLOSE YOUR EYES" printed on it	One point if the patient closes their eyes	1
Writing	Ask the patient to write a sentence	One point if sentence has a subject, a verb, and makes sense	1
Drawing	Ask the patient to copy a pair of intersecting pentagons onto a piece of paper	One point if the figure has ten corners and two intersecting lines	1
	A score of 24 or above is considered normal		30

Table 1. *Folstein's Mini Mental Status Examination*

Age	Must be correct
Time	Without looking at watch/clock; correct to nearest hour
42 East Street	Give this address. Check registration. Check memory at end of test.
Month	Exact
Year	Exact, except in Jan/Feb when previous year OK
Name of place	If not in hospital ask type of place or area of town
Date of birth	Exact
Start of WW1	Exact
Name of present monarch/president	Exact
Count backwards from 20 to 1	Can prompt with the first few numbers, but no further prompts, patient can hesitate and self correct but no other errors
Score 8-10	Normal
Score 7	Probably abnormal
Score < 6	Abnormal

Table 2. *Abbreviated Mental Test score. One point for each correct answer.*

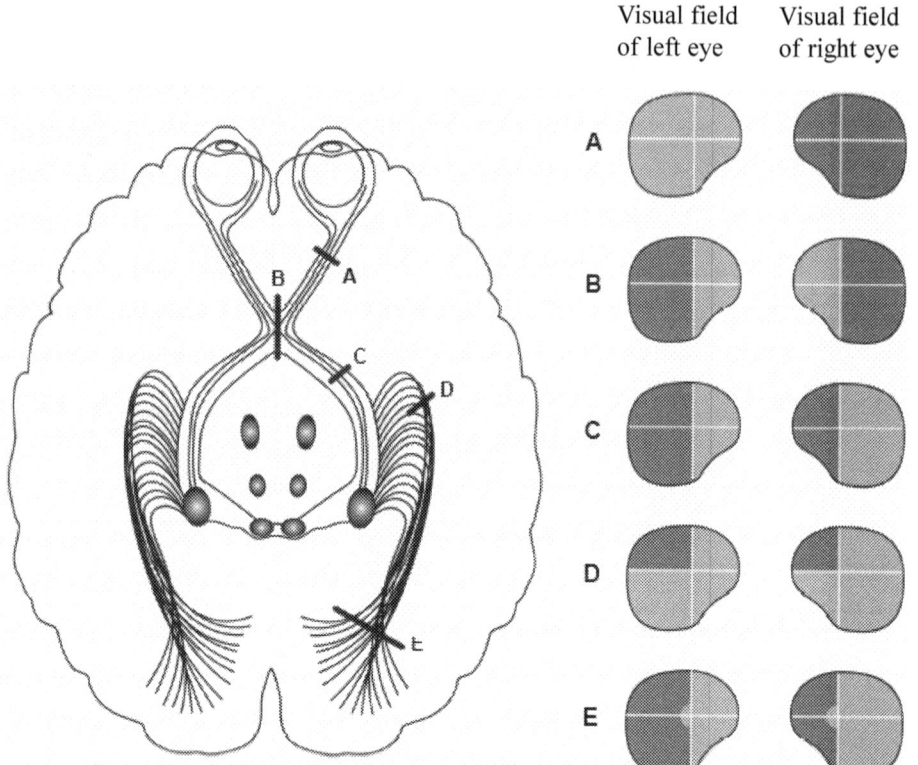

Figure 1. *Visual field deficits according to the site of the compression - A. complete vision loss in right eye, B. bitemporal hemianopia, C. left homonomous hemianopia, D. left upper quadrant hemianopia, E. macular sparing in left homonomous hemianopia. It is important to note that the images transmitted in the nasal fibers of the optic nerve cross over in the chiasm and that the temporal fibres continue straight backwards. It is also important to note that the lower retinal fibres cross anteriorly and the upper retinal fibres cross posteriorly in the chiasm. The lower retinal fibres carry the upper temporal visual field and the upper retinal fibres carry the lower temporal field. Beyond the lateral geniculate body, the fibres fan out into the optic radiation and the fibres serving the lower nasal retina (the upper temporal field) dip into the temporal lobe. These fibres are called Meyer's loop. Compression of these fibres leads to a contralateral upper quadrantanopia. It will be a homonomous hemianopia since the nasal fibres from the contralateral eye would have crossed over in the chiasm. Visual fields can be assessed by visual confrontation testing. See figure 2. The most sensitive way to do this is to use a red pin because red is the first colour that we experience inability to see when there is compression of the optic nerve.*

It is important to remember that patients can have near normal visual acuity with large deficits in their visual fields. Having tested both visual fields and visual acuity it is now important to perform fundoscopy.

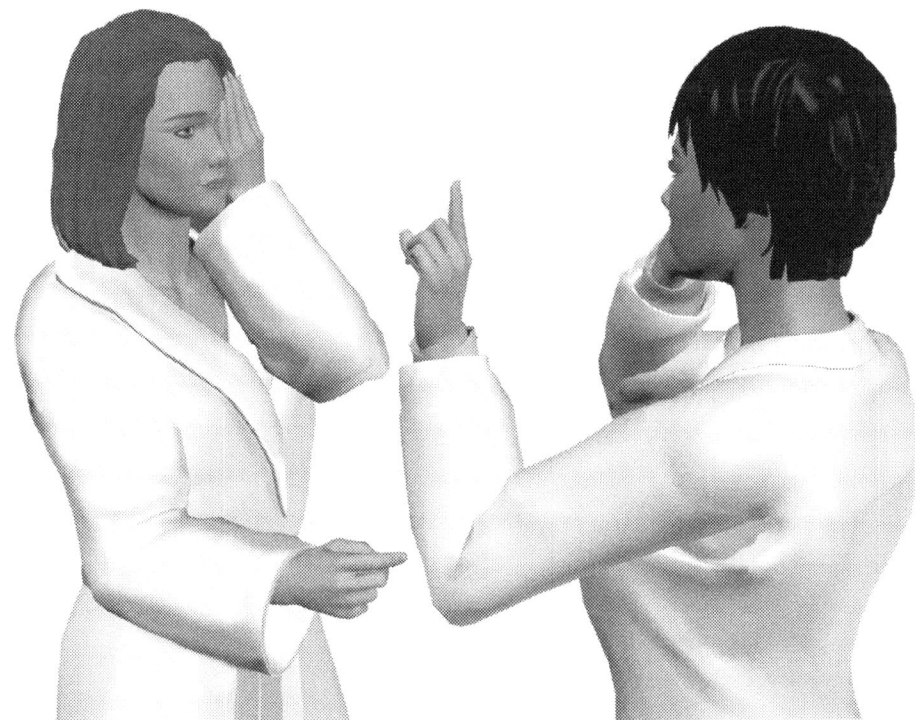

Figure 2. *Visual confrontation testing. Whilst sitting opposite the patient you ask them to occlude their left eye while you occlude your right eye and, using the limits of your own visual field, you test whether the patient has the same extent of visual field. Repeat this with the other eye. Visual fields are recorded as the patient sees them. Therefore the left temporal field will be recorded on the left and the right temporal field on the right.*

Fundoscopy
This is a skill that is learnt only with a lot of practice and it is frequently reported incorrectly. It is important to note that papilloedema (bilateral optic disc swelling) takes 10-14 days to develop and is not present in the patient with acute head injury. It is rather a hallmark of chronic raised intracranial pressure or chronic optic disc pathology. It is frequently said that patients who have no papilloedema are safe to undergo a lumbar puncture without resorting to any cranial imaging. This is incorrect, as a patient who has a large acute subdural haematoma or intracerebral haematoma will not have papilloedema and performing a lumbar puncture on these patients can lead to coning and death.
Papilloedema has four stages. See table 3.

CN III, IV, VI
These three nerves work together to move the eyeball around in its socket. The third cranial nerve has the added function of pupil constriction and carries sympathetic fibres that mediate eyelid elevation. Most of the muscles of the eyeball are supplied by the third cranial nerve, but the *lateral rectus* is supplied by the sixth cranial nerve and the *superior oblique* by the fourth cranial nerve. This causes a patient with a third nerve palsy to have an eyeball which looks downwards and outwards because of the unopposed pull of the *lateral rectus* and *superior oblique muscles*. In cases of *lateral rectus* palsy, the eyeball loses the ability to look laterally. In an isolated fourth nerve palsy, the patient develops diplopia on looking outwards and downwards.

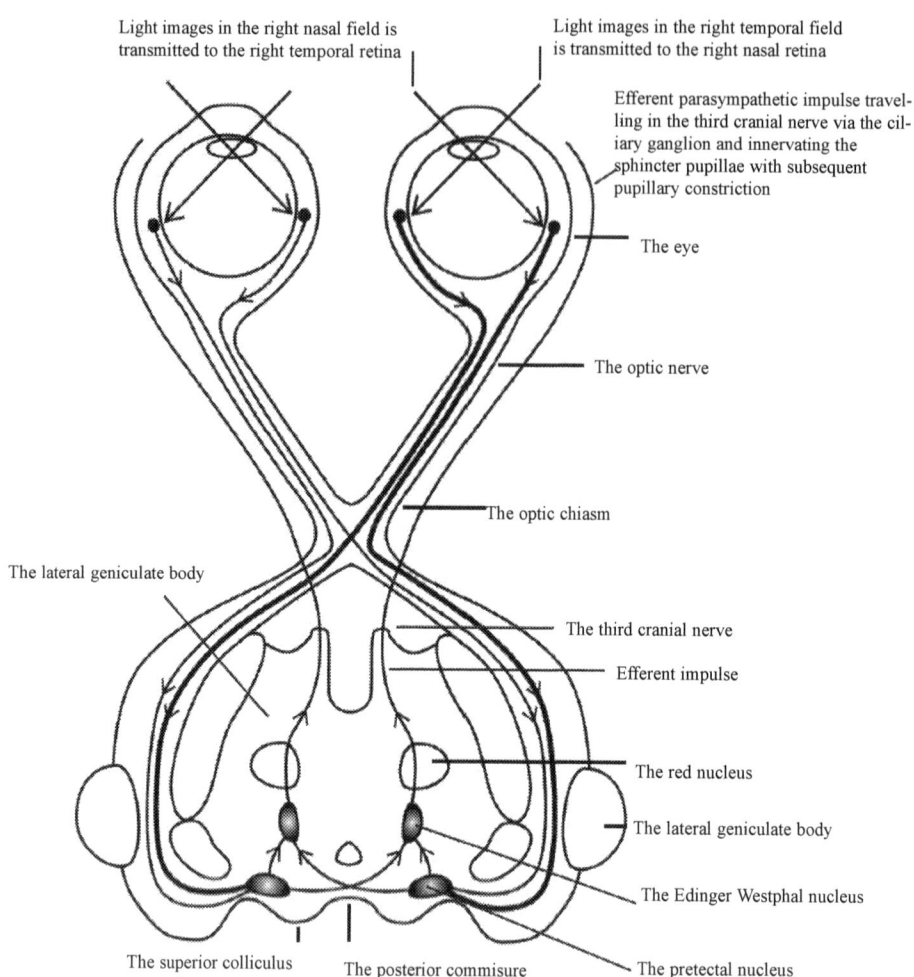

Figure 3. *Pupillary light reflex - pupillary constriction is a parasympathetic function and is mediated by the Edinger-Westphal nuclei. Light impulses travel back in the second cranial nerve and in the brain stem at the level of superior colliculus bilaterally innervates the Edinger-Westphal nuclei. Efferent impulses then travel forwards in both third cranial nerves and therefore light shone into one eye activates constriction in both eyes.*

The *superior oblique* pulls the eye downwards and medially as it acts by hooking around the trochlea and the *inferior rectus* pulls the eye down and laterally. In a patient with fourth cranial nerve palsy, downward gaze results in unopposed action of the *inferior rectus* pulling the affected eye downwards and outwards. Downward gaze therefore precipitates or worsens diplopia. Pupillary constriction is a parasympathetic function and is mediated by the Edinger-Westphal nuclei. Light impulses travel back in the second cranial nerve and in the brain stem at the level of superior colliculus bilaterally innervates the Edinger-Westphal nuclei. Efferent impulses then travel forwards in both third cranial nerves and therefore light shone into one eye activates constriction in both eyes, see figure 3.

Stage one	There is decreased drainage of the veins of the optic nerve and this leads to the veins swelling and becoming tortuous. An experienced observer will also be able to see decreased venous pulsation
Stage two	The optic discs swell and, where the vessels of the optic disc in the normal situation have an acute posterior kink plunging into the optic discs, they now stop at the margin of the disc. The discs frequently changes colour from a pale yellow to pink as this occurs
Stage three	The disc margins swell more and become increasingly indistinct and blurred
Stage four	There is even more swelling of the discs with obvious elevation and scattered haemorrhages frequently seen

Table 3. *Grades of papilloedema*

If there is compression or dysfunction of the afferent pathway of the pupillary reflex (second cranial nerve) this will lead to a Marcus Gunn pupil: light falling on the affected pupil will lead to a larger pupil than when light falls on the unaffected pupil. This is due to the ipsilateral input to the Edinger-Westphal nucleus being weaker (because of the damage to the afferent pathway) than when light is shone into the contralateral eye with the unaffected optic nerve (consensual light reflex). This is demonstrated by swinging a flashlight between the two eyes and seeing a slight dilatation when the light falls directly on the affected eye. Compression of the efferent pathway (third cranial nerve), causes dysfunction of pupil constriction and that leads to a persistently dilated pupil. The pupillary constrictor fibres lie quite superficially in the third nerve and a hallmark of external compression is that of pupillary dilatation. The third nerve also carries sympathetic fibres which innervate the superior tarsal muscles and assist eye opening. Thus a patient with an external compressive third nerve lesion will have a dilated pupil, ptosis and a downward and outward deviated eye (ophthalmoplegia). Pupillary dilatation is a sympathetic activity and is initiated in the hypothalamus with the signals descending in the spinal cord to the level of T1. At the level of T1, the white rami of the nerve roots of C8 and T1 pass through the cervical sympathetic ganglion. Impulses travel from there in sympathetic nerves into the cranial cavity on the surface of the carotid artery and arrive at the pupil via a branch of the ophthalmic artery. When there is dysfunction of the sympathetic system it leads to ptosis because of the decreased innervation of the tarsal muscles, pupillary constriction due to a loss of pupillary dilatation and loss of facial sweating due to autonomic dysfunction. This is called Horner's syndrome and is easily remembered by the rhyme "ptosis, myosis and anhydrosis." The pupillary abnormality is best demonstrated by taking the patient into a darkened room. In normal circumstances, both pupils will dilate in a darkened room but in a patient with Horner's syndrome, the affected pupil will remain constricted.

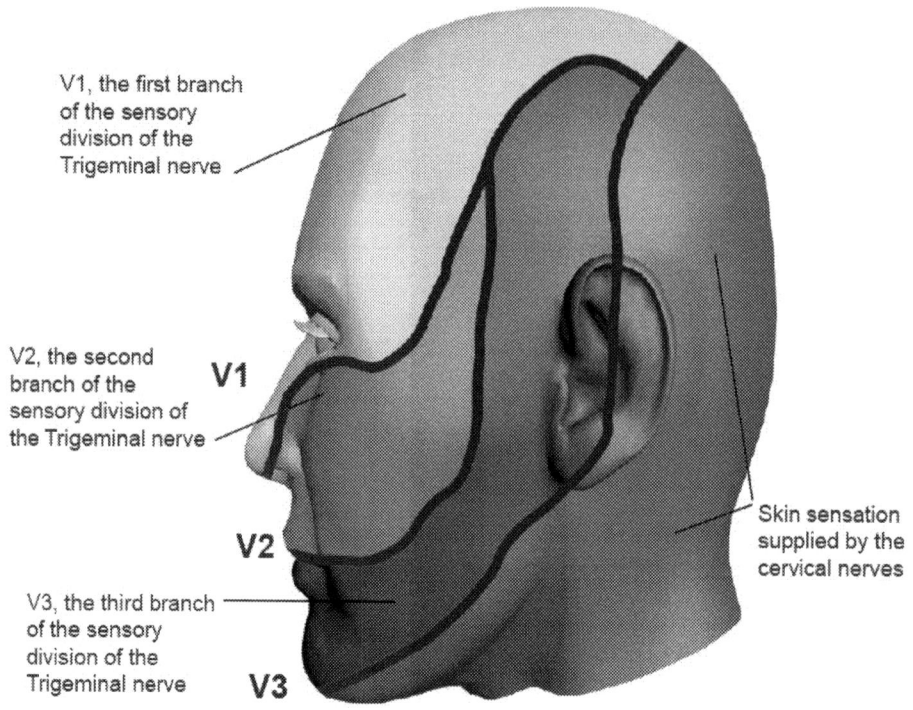

Figure 4. *Distribution of the Trigeminal nerve's sensory divisions. Note that the sensation in front of the tragus is supplied by the 7th and 9th cranial nerves (not demonstrated)*

CN V
The first division of the fifth cranial nerve accompanies the third, fourth and sixth cranial nerves through the cavernous sinus and these four nerves are frequently compromised together by lesions in the cavernous sinus. The fifth cranial nerve's largest component is the sensory division but it also has a motor division that serves mastication. It is assessed by testing sensation over the face and by testing corneal sensation (first division) and the jaw jerk. It is important to realise that the first division of the fifth cranial nerve actually supplies sensation as far back as the coronal suture, but does not supply the jaw line. See figure 4.

CN VII
The seventh cranial nerve is almost purely made up of motor fibres and supplies the muscles of the face. The facial nerve has a supranuclear input which supplies the ipsilateral side of the face and also a reflex component that is primarily concerned with reflex eye closure and has no cortical component. Both eyes will shut if there is danger to either individual eye and therefore there is dual innervation of both sides of the forehead. If there is dysfunction of the cortical innervation (supranuclear innervation) this leads to deficient lower face muscle function and intact upper face function. The seventh cranial nerve also has a small sensory function and carries sensation from the external auditory canal and taste sensation from the anterior two-thirds of the tongue via the chorda tympani.

CN VIII
The vestibulocochlear nerve consists of the vestibular nerve and the cochlear nerve. The vestibular nerve serves balance and the cochlear nerve hearing. Hearing can be tested by rubbing your fingers next to the patient's ears and determining whether they can hear that or, alternatively, whispering numbers in their ears and asking the patient to relay which numbers

have been whispered. Weber and Rinne's tests are useful in distinguishing between conductive and sensory neural deafness. Weber's test consists of placing a vibrating tuning fork on the patient's vertex and asking if the patient feels or hears it best on one side or the other. A patient with no abnormalities will experience no difference. In cases with unilateral neurosensory hearing loss, the hearing will be best in the normal ear, while in cases of a unilateral conductive hearing loss, it is best heard in the abnormal ear. In Rinne's test, bone conduction (placing the tuning fork on the mastoid process) is compared to air conduction (placing the tuning fork in front of but not touching the pinna). Normally, air conduction is greater than bone conduction. In cases of partial neurosensory hearing loss, air conduction is still greater than bone conduction but in cases of conduction hearing loss bone conduction will be greater than air conduction. It is sometimes difficult to remember which test does what but I remember Weber's test as being the one where you put the tuning fork on top of somebody's head by the fact that a 'W' looks a bit like a crown.

CN IX, X, XI

These nerves share the same motor nucleus (nucleus ambiguus) and all exit the skull through the jugular foramen. The **glossopharyngeal nerve (IX)** is the main afferent pathway of the gag reflex and also, along with the seventh cranial nerve, supplies some sensation in the external auditory canal and conveys taste, in this case, from the posterior third of the tongue. The only function that we routinely test is the gag reflex and the efferent pathway of the gag reflex is the tenth cranial nerve **(vagus)**. The tenth cranial nerve also supplies motor fibres to the muscles of the palate. Testing the ninth and tenth nerves together then consists of testing the gag reflex and also testing the patient's palatal muscles by asking them to open their mouth widely and saying "aaaahh" whilst using a light to illuminate the back of the mouth. If there is a palsy of the vagus, there will be asymmetry of the palate and a left-sided nerve palsy will cause the intact muscles on the right-hand side to pull the palate over to the right and vice-versa. Having a depressed gag reflex can either be because of dysfunction in the ninth or tenth cranial nerve. Patients with a ninth nerve palsy will usually have normal palatal function. The gag is tested by stimulating the uvula and posterior pharynx with a tongue depressor. The tenth cranial nerve also supplies the larynx and a vagal or recurrent laryngeal nerve palsy causes ipsilateral vocal cord paralysis and a hoarse voice.

The **spinal accessory nerve (XI)** originates in a nucleus in the spinal cord and leaves the spinal cord through the cervical branches supplying the *sternocleidomastoid and trapezius muscles* on the same side. The unusual feature of this nerve is that the higher control is not crossed and a right-sided lesion will therefore lead to a right-sided nerve dysfunction. The *sternocleidomastoid muscle* pulls the patient's head towards the opposite side and right *sternocleidomastoid muscle* (right eleventh nerve) function is therefore tested by asking the patient to look towards the left against resistance and simultaneously palpating the muscles on the right-hand side. A patient with a right hemisphere lesion will not be able to look towards the left-hand side and if we remember the anatomy of the second cranial nerve, they will have inattention of the left visual field. Therefore patients with extensive right hemisphere damage will not be aware of the left-hand side and will not be able to look towards the left-hand side.

CN XII

The twelfth cranial nerve supplies the motor function of the tongue and is tested by both observation and active movement. Observing the tongue lying in the floor of the mouth with the patient's mouth open will demonstrate any fasciculation if present. The patient is then asked to push the tongue out of their mouth and move it from side to side. If there is a palsy, the stronger intact muscles will push the tongue towards the affected weaker side and therefore the tongue will deviate towards the affected side (whereas in the case of a tenth nerve palsy, the palate will pull away from the affected side). This can be remembered by the fact that the tongue muscles push out and the palatal muscles pull up.

CN I	Usually reserved for cases where the patient reports a decrease in olfaction
CN II	Visual confrontation, acuity and fundoscopy
CN III, IV, VI	Eye movements
CN V	Facial sensation
CN VII	Facial movements
CN VIII	Rubbing your fingers next to the ear (Rinne, Weber)
CN IX - XII	Gag reflex, palatal function, shoulder and neck movements and looking at tongue movements

Table 4. *Examination of the cranial nerves*

Examination of the motor system
The left hemisphere controls the right-hand side of the body and vice versa. The motor system is made up of two parts: the main controlling pyramidal system (named after the pyramids in the medulla oblongata) and the extrapyramidal system which modulates the pyramidal system and does not cross over. Motor signals are generated in the cortex and then travel via the corona radiata and the internal capsule down to the brainstem. They cross over in the medulla oblongata to the opposite side to control motor movement. The extrapyramidal system modulates the actions of the pyramidal system based on proprioception and feedback via the cerebellum. In a hemispheric deficit there is dysfunction of the motor system on the whole of the contralateral side. A large left hemispheric infarct will produce a paralysis of the right side of the face, the right arm and the right leg. Because the reflex arc of the spinal cord is independent of cerebral input, patients who are completely paralysed will still have intact reflexes. Reflexes are however modulated by higher input and if there is dysfunction anywhere in the brain or the spinal cord the effect downstream of that will be a decrease in modulation of the reflex activity. Therefore patients who have a left hemisphere infarct will have spastic right arm and leg reflexes due to non-modulated reflex arc activity. This is also true if the cause of the paralysis is in the spinal cord which will lead to decreased muscle power below the level of the lesion and increase in the reflexes (hyperreflexia). This is extremely useful in delineating the level of the pathology. Somebody who has damage to the spinal cord at C6 level will have increased reflexes below the level of C6 as well as weakness below that level with normal power and reflexes above that level. The rule for establishing the level of spinal pathology is that at the level of injury there will be decreased reflexes and weakness (lower motor neurone signs) and below the level there will be weakness and increased reflexes (upper motor neurone signs). Lesions distal to the anterior horn cells in the spinal cord lead to lower motor neurone signs (decreased or absent reflexes and weakness). Patients who have only dysfunction of a nerve root might have a radiculopathy and the myotome as well as the dermatome served by this nerve will show dysfunction. For instance somebody with a centrally herniated intervertebral disc (slipped disc) at the L4/5 lumbar level might have a L5 radiculopathy which, if it only involves the sensory component will produce numbness on the dorsum of the foot. If it is severe and also involves the motor component, they will have difficulty with extension (dorsiflexion) of their ankle. When examining the motor system you have to test the tone of the muscles, the muscle power (table 6) and reflexes (table 5).

Description	Score
Absent	-4
Just elicitable	-3
Low	-2
Moderately low	-1
Normal	0
Brisk	1
Very brisk	2
Exhaustible clonus	3
Continuous clonus	4

Table 5. *Mayo Clinic scale for tendon reflex assessment*

Score	Muscle Response
0	No Movement
1	Muscle belly moves but the joint does not move
2	Joint moves with gravity eliminated
3	Joint moves against gravity
4	Joint moves against gravity and some resistance
5	Full strength

Table 6. *MRC Scale for Grading Muscle Strength*

Extrapyramidal system (cerebellar function)
Pathology in the cerebellum causes ipsilateral deficits so that an infarct of the left cerebellum will lead to left-sided weakness and hypotonia. It is important to note that extrapyramidal weakness is not associated with hyperreflexia. Pathology causes a dysfunctional proprioception feedback system and will cause the limbs on the ipsilateral side to be ataxic. Lesions of the vermis, on the other hand, will lead to truncal ataxia. Limb ataxia can be tested by checking the patient for past pointing with the ability to do the finger-nose test and testing for the presence of dysdiadocokinesia. In the lower limbs ataxia can be tested by asking the patient to tap his foot on the floor or to do the heel-to-shin test. Another marker of possible cerebellar pathology is nystagmus.

Muscles	Root Levels	Clinical
Trapezius	C3-C4	Shrug shoulders
Deltoid	C5-C6	Abduct shoulder
Biceps	C5-C6	Flex elbow
Triceps	C6-C8	Extend elbow
Wrist extensors	C6-C7	Extend wrist
Wrist flexors	C6-T1	Flex wrist
Hand intrinsic muscles	C8-T1	Spread fingers
Opponens pollicis and digiti minimi	C8-T1	Make "o" with thumb and 5th finger
Iliopsoas	**L2**-L3	Flex hip
Quadriceps	**L3**-L4	Extend knee
Hamstrings	L5-S1	Flex knee
Gluteus maximus	S1-S2	Extend hip
Tibialis anterior	L4-L5	Dorsiflex foot
Tibialis posterior	L4-5	Invert foot
Peroneii	L5-**S1**	Evert foot
Extensor hallucis longus	**L5**	Extend (dorsiflex) great toe
Gastrocnemius	**S1**-S2	Plantar flexion

Table 7. *Myotomes*

Tendon	Root
Bicep reflex	C5/6
Brachioradialis reflex	C6
Triceps	C7
Patella (knee) reflex	L4
Achilles (ankle) reflex	S1

Table 8. *Deep tendon reflexes*

Gait

The last part of evaluation of the motor system is to test the patient's gait. A lot can be learned from a patient's gait. Patients with severe lower back pain and radicular pain will have a type of gait where they put less pressure on the affected side and walk with a limp. This is called an antalgic type of gait. Patients who have suffered cerebrovascular accidents, often have a fixed flexion of their upper limb and a straight, outstretched leg with a plantar-flexed foot which causes them to walk by circumducting the affected leg. They do this by swinging the stiff leg out and around before putting it down. Where there is cerebellar pathology the patient may have a general unsteadiness due to limb ataxia. Patients who are myelopathic have a stiff, spastic gait and frequently shuffle along.

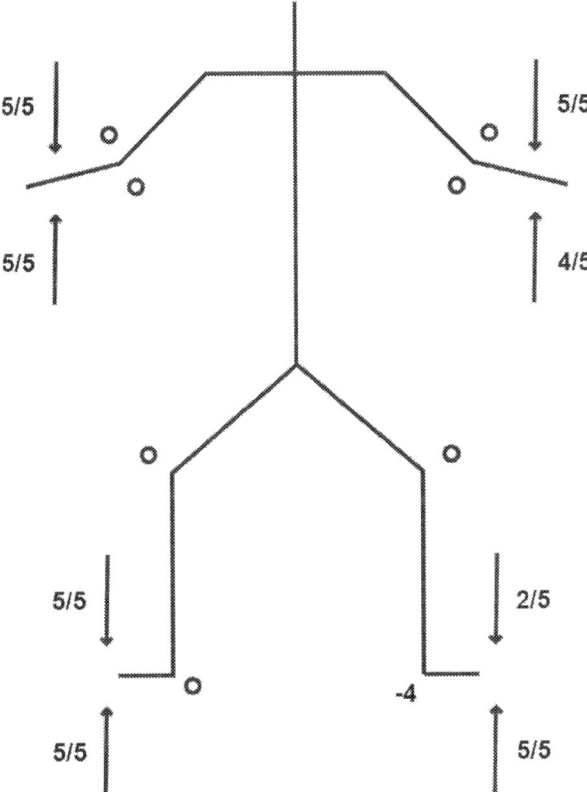

Figure 6. *Notation of the motor system examination. The motor strength (Table 6) and reflexes (Table 5) should be noted on a visual chart as above.*

Romberg
Following assessment of gait you may want to do a Romberg's test. Romberg's test is based on the fact that we need at least 2 out of 3 senses to be able to stand unaided (proprioception, vestibular function, vision). If patients close their eyes and they have a deficit in either their vestibular function or proprioception, they will fall over. This is, however, not a very specific test.

Overview of the motor examination
The suggested sequence for examining the motor system is as follows:
Ask the patient to hold their arms stretched out in front of them with palms upward facing. Ask them to close their eyes. Any subtle weakness will result in a drift of the arm on the weak side. Now ask the patient to open their eyes, turn their palms downwards towards the floor and to make piano playing movements with their fingers. If they can do this, you have successfully screened for subtle motor weakness. You have also tested proprioception and fine motor movements and therefore have tested both pyramidal and extrapyramidal systems. This can be followed up by testing tone in all 4 limbs, one at a time and then testing motor function in all the myotomes. The last step is to test the reflexes. Examination for the motor system should be noted down as demonstrated in figure 6.

Examination of the sensory system
When testing the sensory system it is always very important to ask the patient whether they are aware of any abnormal sensation. If they are not then it is unlikely that you will find any deficit. In testing for sensation it is important to test the different sensory modalities (light touch, temperature, pain and joint position sense).

If you are testing for pain it usually negates the necessity to test for temperature sensation as well, except in patients where we have reason to suspect hydromyelia or syringomyelia where the loss of temperature sensation is quite typical. We therefore effectively have 3 modalities that we test for – proprioception, the fibres of which are located in the posterior part of the spinal cord, light touch, the fibres of which are located in the anterior part of the spinal cord and pain, the fibres of which are located in the lateral part of the spinal cord. Light touch can be tested by running your fingertips or cotton wool lightly along the patient's skin. Pain sensation is tested with a pinprick. Proprioception and joint position sense is tested by moving the patient's toes, feet, fingers or hands with their eyes closed. When testing pain sensation it is important to realise that the pain fibres cross over in the spinal cord and not at the brain stem unlike the other fibres. Therefore a lesion that is restricted to only one half of the spinal cord will lead to ipsilateral proprioceptive and light touch abnormalities, and contralateral pain sensation abnormalities below the affected spinal level (dermatome). This is the basis for the Brown-Séquard syndrome.

It is important not to fall in the C4/T2 trap and to realise that the dermatomes on the chest for C4 and T2 are close to each other and therefore a C4 lesion can be mistaken for a thoracic lesion if the sensation in the arms is not tested. Somebody who is numb from just above the level of their nipples downwards and therefore has a sensory level just above their nipples might have a T3/4 lesion but, if you were to examine their arms that contain the cervical dermatomes and find that they were numb as well, you would have to conclude that this was actually a cervical rather than a thoracic lesion. See figure 7 for the anatomical pattern of dermatomes. Another type of sensory deficit is a cortical sensory deficit and patients with lesions in their parietal lobe might have a deficiency in two point discrimination and discrimination of objects.

Examination of the comatose patient
Examination of the comatose patient is restricted to testing the pupillary reactivity, the Glasgow Coma Scale, the presence of a paresis or paralysis and the patient's reflexes including pathological reflexes (Babinski). The Glasgow Coma Scale is made up of the motor response, the verbal response and eye opening.

The motor response comprises 6 points. See table 8. The notation for a patient's GCS is as follows: GCS (total score)/15, M (score), V (score), E (score). Patients who are intubated have an annotated T added to indicate intubation (GCS 7/15 T). Following notation of the GCS, the pupillary activity is then noted and the term "PEARL" can be used which stands for pupils equal and reactive to light. Following notation of the GCS and the pupillary activity, the focal deficit must be noted down for paresis or paralysis of any of the limbs. Verbal response is scored out of 5. It needs to be remembered that someone who has a lesion focally in Broca's area will not be able to speak properly and will therefore drop several points on the Glasgow Coma Scale. Therefore somebody with a Glasgow Coma Scale of 11/15 may be completely awake and orientated,but completely aphasic, see table 9 for a summary of the verbal response. Eye opening response is scored out of 4. See table 10 for a summary of the eye opening response.

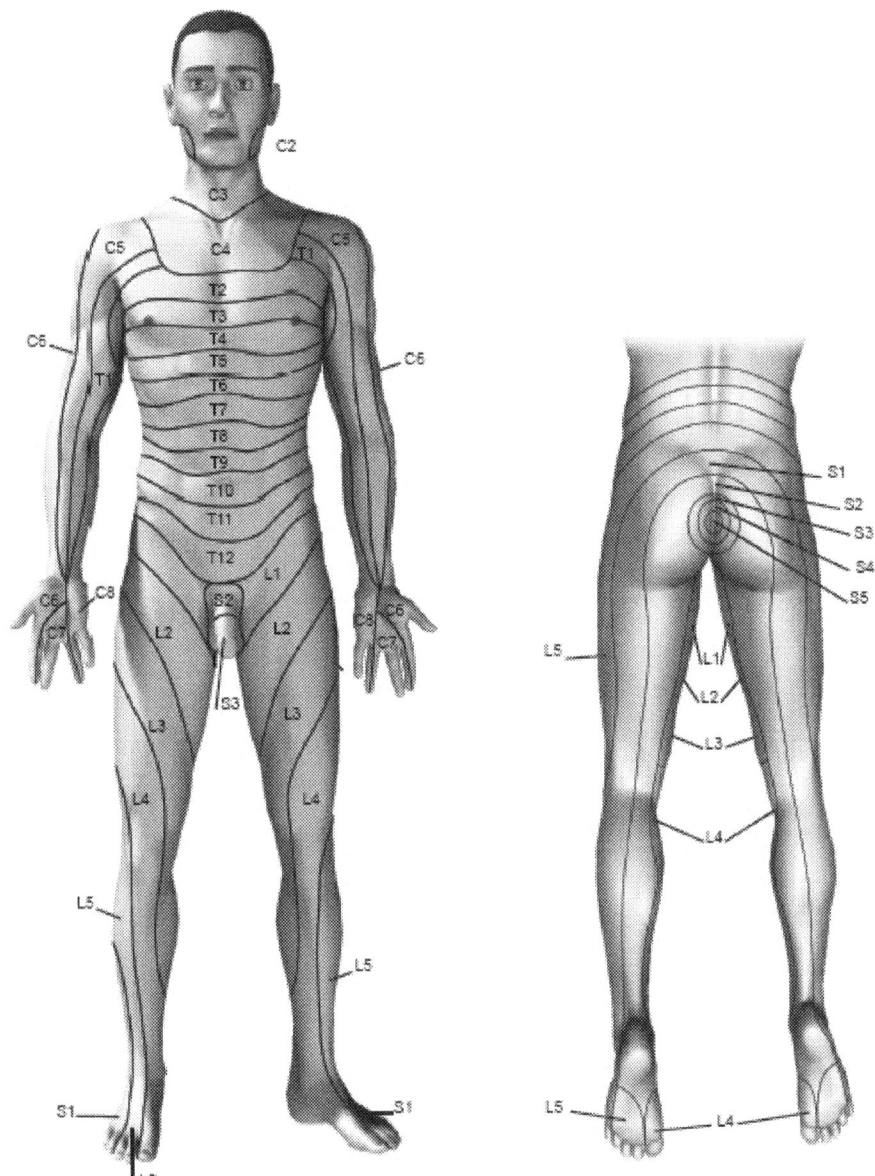

Figure 7. *Human dermatomes*

6/6	Ability to follow commands which requires a rather sophisticated train of events to occur in the nervous system
5/6	The awareness and localisation of painful stimuli. Painful stimulus on the chest wall will therefore lead to the patient grasping your hand and even trying to pull it away
4/6	The patient is aware of the pain or threat and attempts to localise it but cannot. Patients who flex their limbs but are unable to localise the painful stimulus.
3/6	The patient's arms are spasmodically fully flexed next to the body. This is an action that has no reliance on cognition of the cortex and is therefore called decorticate posturing
2/6	The arms are spasmodically extended on either side of the body; the legs are also spastic and extended. This is a final reflex stage that does not rely on the cerebrum at all and so it is called decerebrate posturing. Posturing, both decorticate and decerebrate carry a poor prognosis
1/6	No motor response. Therefore somebody who has even a flicker of movement will get a score of 2/6

Table 8. *Motor response (GCS)*

5/5	Patient is fully orientated to person, time and place
4/5	Confused speech
3/5	Words only
2/5	Sounds only
1/5	No sound whatsoever

Table 9. *Verbal response (GCS)*

4/4	The patient spontaneously opens the eyes
3/4	The patient opens the eyes to verbal stimuli
2/4	The patient opens the eyes to painful stimuli
1/4	The patient does not open the eyes at all

Table 10. *Eye opening response*

3

CRANIAL IMAGING

Contents

Introduction
CT scans
Tissue densities
MRI scans
Physics
Sequences
Tissue intensities
Blood changes with time on MR scans
An approach to reading scans and radiological anatomy
Hydrocephalus and ventriculomegaly

Trauma
Skull fractures
Diffuse Brain Injury
Intracerebral haemorrhage
Extra axial collections

Brain Tumours
Primary brain tumours
(Low grade) astrocytoma
Anaplastic astrocytoma
Glioblastoma Multiforme
Pilocytic astrocytoma
Oligodendroglioma
Ependymoma
Meningioma
Primary central nervous system lymphoma

Intracranial cyst-like lesions
Dermoid cyst
Epidermoid cyst
Colloid cyst of the third ventricle
Arachnoid cyst

Pituitary region tumours
Microadenomas
Macroadenomas
Craniopharyngiomas

Neuronal tumours
Central neurocytomas

Pineal region tumours
Germinoma
Pineal parenchymal tumours

Tumours of the posterior fossa
Hemangioblastoma
Medulloblastoma
Astrocytoma

Skull base tumours
Chordoma
Vestibular schwannoma

Metastatic tumours

Vascular Pathology
Arterial infarct
Venous infarct
Spontaneous haemorrhage
Subarachnoid haemorrhage (aneurysmal)
Parenchymal hypertensive haemorrhage
Vascular anomalies
Arteriovenous Malformation
Cavernous malformation
Venous angioma

Infection
Empyema
Cerebritis
Abscess

Introduction

I remember being amazed at the skill of the neurosurgical registrars in reading CT and MRI scans when I was a trauma doctor. A scan was quite a frightening investigation to me and I was unsure how to evaluate them. I think this is probably true for many doctors. The scan can however be an exceedingly straightforward test to read since the brain is a relatively symmetrical structure and it is therefore quite easy to pick up asymmetry denoting underlying abnormalities. Once you can identify the normal anatomy, there are a few simple rules to follow to lead you to a differential diagnosis. Even the most experienced physicians and radiologists can only take a diagnosis up to a certain level and will mostly end up saying that "this is most probably lesion x but it could also be lesion y or z". For me, the cranial scan is a clinical test in the sense that it has much less relevance if not interpreted in the context of the clinical setting. The patient's history and examination should really have brought you quite close to a diagnosis in the first place and should have set a differential diagnosis in your mind already. If you combine the history and examination with a few simple rules in this chapter then you should be able to narrow down the diagnosis quite efficiently without needing a great deal of knowledge about neurosurgery.

CT scans

A Computed Tomography scan is a process where ordinary X-rays (tomograms) are fed through a computer (computed - therefore the term computed tomography) to form a 2D or 3D picture. Different tissues have different densities to X-ray penetration and are reported as hypo, iso and hyperdense. Iodine based contrast is used to enhance areas of increased blood flow or capillary leakage which show up as more dense areas on CT scans since these areas have a higher load of radiodense contrast material.

Tissue densities:
There are four shades of grayscale that tissues can have on a CT scan: white, grey, dark grey and black.
White (hyperdense)
Bone
Calcium deposits
Blood (fresh)
Melanin
Contrast enhancement
Grey (isodense)
Brain
Glial tumours
Blood (subacute)
Dark grey (hypodense)
Most fluid is seen as dark grey, quite close to pure black and if there are different densities, it usually indicates deposits within the fluid.
CSF (ventricles, subarachnoid spaces)
Brain oedema
Fat
Dermoid tumours are black due to fatty deposits
Blood (chronic)
Black (hypodense)
Air

Hounsfield units
The pixels that make up a CT scan image are assigned a numerical value and these values can be used to identify the type of tissue shown on the image. These values range between -1000 for air and +1000 for bone and water is designated as 0. Fat generally has a value of -50 and soft tissues a value of +40.

MRI scans

Physics
Magnetic Resonance Imaging is a process where the body's hydrogen atoms are aligned by a strong magnet (the magnetic part) and is then subjected to powerful radio wave frequencies that are used to push them out of alignment. The hydrogen atoms alternately absorb and emit radio wave energy, vibrating backwards and forwards between their magnetised resting state and their agitated state caused by the radio pulses (the "resonance" part of MRI). Depending on how quickly these atoms return to their original state, the computer can deduce what kind of tissue is represented by the signals returned. This is based on the intensities of the returned signal and therefore the tissues are reported as being hypo, iso and hyperintense (compared to *densities* in CT scans). A paramagnetic contrast medium, Gadolinium is used in a similar fashion as iodine-based contrast is used in CT scans.

Sequences
The different imaging techniques generated by the radio frequency pulses are called pulse sequences. They include amongst other, spin-echo, inversion recovery, gradient echo and FLAIR (fluid attenuation inversion recovery) sequences. By changing the scan repetition

time (TR - the time between RF pulses) and the echo time (TE - the time between the RF pulse and recording the MR signal), it is possible to change the sequence. The two main types of MRI sequences that are used are T1 and T2 weighted images. The terms T1 and T2 refer to the relaxation of the excited nuclei to their original alignment after being excited by the radio waves (relaxation times).

A variant T1-weighted image (T1 WI) is the **STIR** (short tau inversion recovery) sequence which removes bright fat that obscures the signal of interest in orbital or spine images, with pathology being conspicuously bright.
Proton density is neither a T1 nor a T2-weighted image (T2 WI) and is designed to minimise the effects of T1 and T2 WI. Proton density is the concentration of protons in the tissue in the form of water and macromolecules.
FLAIR (fluid attenuation inversion recovery) sequences are a variant of T2 WI where normal body water is suppressed to show pathological oedematous tissue, which is conspicuously bright.
T1 WI are useful in delineating anatomy and return high intensity signals in the following tissues:
Fat
Melanin
Subacute blood
Fluids with high protein content
Paramagnetic contrast agents

T2 WI are very sensitive to most types of pathology and tissues that return high intensity signals are:
Fluid collections (CSF, tissue oedema)
Infarcted brain
Demyelination
Infection
Neoplasms (most)

T1 WI and T2 WI
Flowing blood moves through the plane of the imaging and does not remain present long enough for the spinning hydrogen atoms to return their signal and therefore return little or no signal. Flowing blood is therefore dark on both T1 WI and T2 WI and the signal returned is referred to as a flow void. Air, calcification (bone) and fibrous tissue also return little or no signal due to a paucity of mobile protons and appear dark on both sequences.

Tissue intensities
White matter, because of its high lipid and low water content, is hypointense (relative to grey matter) on T2 WI and hyperintense on T1 WI. On the other hand, grey matter has higher water content than white matter and will therefore be less intense on T1 WI and more intense on T2 WI. CSF therefore appears dark on T1 WI and has a very high signal on T2 WI. The pituitary gland and infundibulum appear grey on T1 WI and T2 WI. When disease processes infiltrate the white matter and displace the hydrophobic tissue with more hydrophilic tissue, the intensities decrease on T1 WI and increase on T2 WI. Most brain tumours return decreased signal intensity on T1 WI and increased signal intensity on T2 WI. In general, pathological processes increase the water content of tissues and appear bright on T2 WI and have decreased signal on T1 WI but there are a few important exceptions to this rule:
Blood (subacute) and melanin is intrinsically bright (white) on T1 WI. Tumours with a high nuclear to cytoplasmic ration such as lymphomas and primitive neuroectodermal tumours (PNET) are also iso/ hyperintense on T1 WI. Multiple areas of increased signal intensity on T2 WI raise the suspicion of secondary metastatic disease, demyelination or vascular disease.

Blood changes with time on MR scans
Depends on age of clot
In T1 WI – remember '**B**ig **G**reat **W**hite **B**ear!'
Hyperacute, within hours - **B**lack (hypointense)
Acute stage, less than 3 days - **G**rey (isointense),
Subacute stage, 3 to 14 days - **W**hite (hyperintense),
Chronic stage, more than 14 days - **B**lack (hypointense)

In T2 WI – remember '**B**ear, **W**hat **B**ear?'
Acute stage – **B**lack (hypointense)
Subacute – **W**hite (hyperintense)
Subacute stage and chronic stages – **B**lack (hypointense)

An approach to reading scans and radiological anatomy

Both MRI and CT scan images are presented as slices through different parts of the skull and brain. On the scan there is usually a scout or survey image that shows a lateral view of the head and neck with lines that have corresponding numbers on them. This is a road map to the slices that can be seen in the rest of the scan. Following the road map indicates which of the axial slices go where in the 3-dimensional anatomic model, see figure 1. About a quarter of the way down through the cranium the ventricles start to appear. They can be discerned from the brain, which is grey, by the fact that they are darker in colour, and nearly pitch black on CT scans and T1 WI and hyperintense on T2 WI. The ventricular system consists of a pair of lateral ventricles, the third ventricle and a fourth ventricle. The third and fourth ventricles are connected by the aqueduct of Sylvius, which we can see on a MRI scan, but not a CT scan. The lateral ventricles have frontal and occipital horns and, in cases of hydrocephalus, we can see the temporal horns of the lateral ventricles. The third ventricle is usually slit-like but in cases of hydrocephalus and obstruction will become round and distended. The fourth ventricle is in the posterior fossa below the level of the tentorium cerebelli and is usually sickle-shaped. The bone of the cranium is brilliant white on CT scans. Just like ordinary X-rays, the tissues that are relatively impenetrable to the rays are recorded as white on the final film and tissues that allow the rays to pass through are darker in colour.

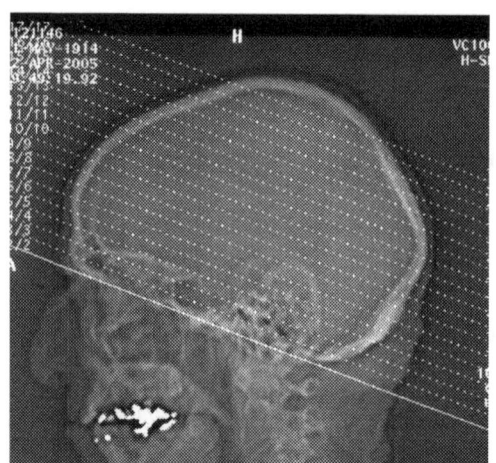

Figure 1. *Note how the CT scan contains a topogram or scout view in the top left hand corner which is a lateral view of the skull with lines running through it. These lines have numbers and the slices that follow are axial images and have corresponding numbers on them so that we can identify through which part of the cranium they were taken. The bottom slices are small and have a lot of bone and very little brain in them as they are in the uppermost part of the cranium and as we travel through the brain, and move up the scan, the slices become progressively larger.*

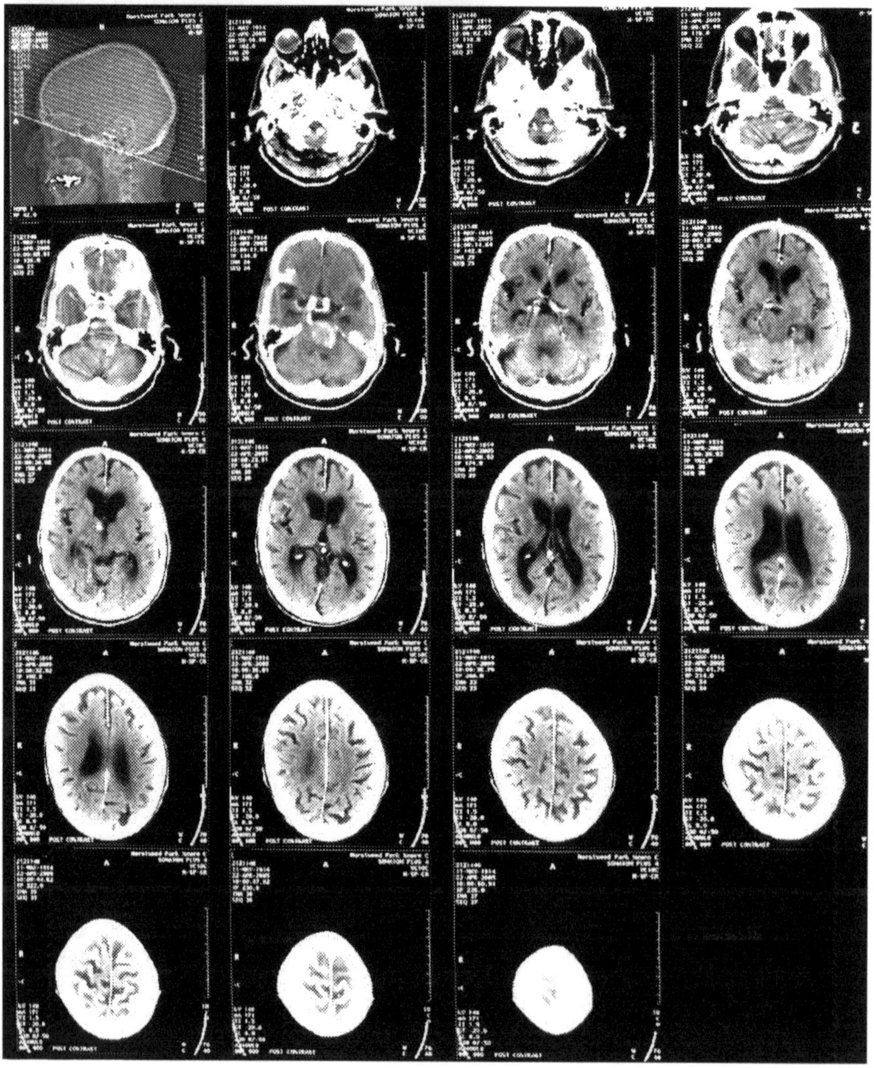

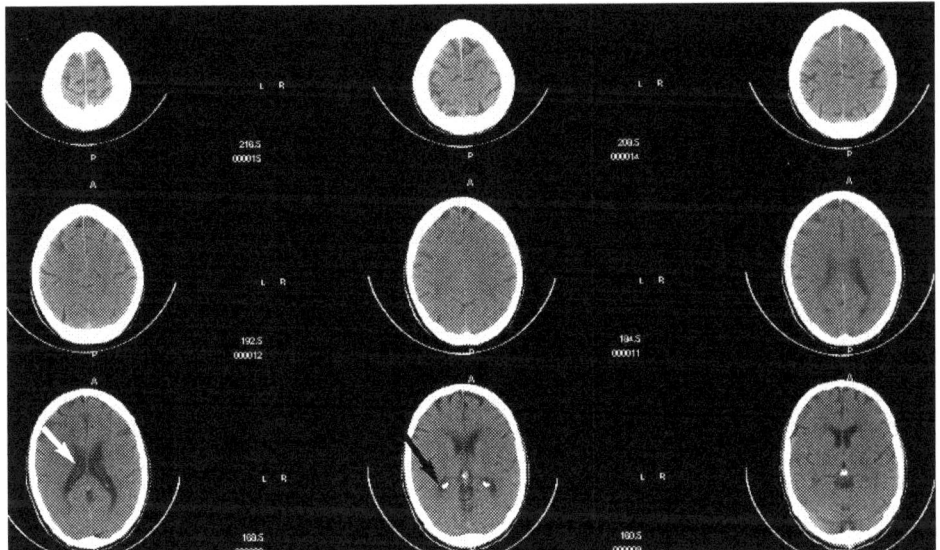

Figure 2. *Note how the size of the images changes as the cuts move from top to bottom through the cranial space. In this electronic image, the uppermost images correspond to the top of the cranium as opposed to the other way around on the hard copy seen in figure 1. Note the lateral ventricles as denoted by the white arrow and the white of the calcified choroid plexus in the trigone of the right lateral ventricle as denoted by the black arrow*

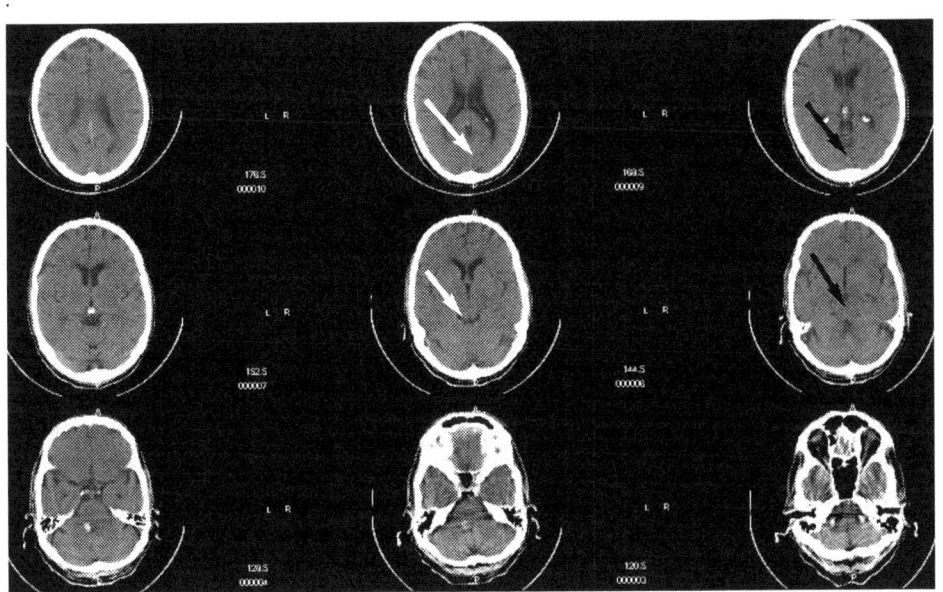

Figure 3. *Note the falx (top white arrow), denoting the supratentorial space and how on the next slice, the falx disappears and the top of the posterior fossa is demonstrated (top black arrow). Note the basal cisterns as demonstrated by the bottom white arrow and the brainstem as denoted by the bottom black arrow. The basal cisterns have a fluid density as they contain CSF.*

Bone is dark on MRI (T1 WI and T2 WI) because of the calcium deposited in it. At the edges of the brain adjacent to the bone, there are fluid-filled spaces, the subarachnoid spaces, and these are the same colour as the ventricles (dark on CT scan and T1 WI and white on T2 WI) since both contain CSF.

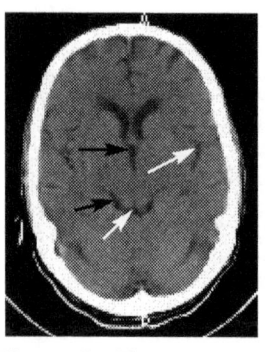

Figure 4. *This is an uncontrasted axial CT scan. The top black arrow indicates the slit like third ventricle, the bottom black arrow the ambient cistern, the bottom white arrow the quadrigeminal cistern and the top white arrow the sylvian fissure.*

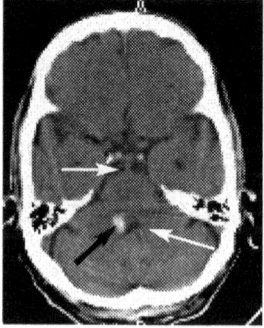

Figure 5. *This is an uncontrasted axial CT scan. The top arrows shows the pre pontine cistern and the bottom arrow the fourth ventricle, which in this case contains fresh blood (black arrow).*

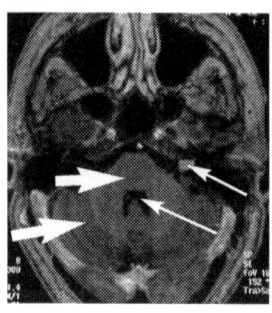

Figure 6. *This is a contrast enhanced axial T1 WI. The top thick arrow demonstrates the pons and the bottom thick arrow demonstrates the cerebellum. The top thin arrow demonstrates a small intracanalicular vestibular schwannoma in the cerebellopontine angle and the bottom thin arrow demonstrates the sickle shaped fourth ventricle.*

Just posterior to the third ventricle, the brain stem can be seen with the basal cisterns around it. These consist of the prepontine, ambient and quadrigeminal cisterns. The supratentorial space is separated from the infratentorial space by the tentorium cerebelli. In the supratentorial space you will see the two cerebral hemispheres separated by the falx cerebrum. Immediately below the level of the tentorium, the falx is no longer visible and this is the anatomical space of the posterior fossa in which the cerebellum is housed. The cerebellum abuts the brain stem and the area between the brainstem and the cerebellum is called the cerebellopontine angle.

Some of the different structures of the brain seen on scans are the parenchyma consisting of white matter and grey matter, the subarachnoid spaces including the basal cisterns, the ventricular system, the substance of the cerebellum and then the bony vault and skull base surrounding the brain. T1 WI are excellent for demonstrating normal anatomy. In evaluating a patient's radiology, it is important to make sure that you know how many films have been done. A patient may have several sets of films; there may be three CT scan films, one for evaluation of the bone in which only bone windows were done and the brain had been factored out, one where soft tissue had been factored in without contrast and one where soft tissue had been factored in post contrast enhancement. The MRI will usually consist of several types of sequences with T2 WI and pre and post contrast T1 WI being the most common. The MRI will consist of not only axial cuts but also coronal and sagittal cuts. When putting the scans up onto the viewer, look in the right upper corner of each of the small images and identify the name of the patient. Ensure the scan is orientated the correct way around (if the name of the patient is not back to front or upside down, you are correct in your orientation). Ensure that the films you are looking at are for the correct scan date. Then try to find a "c" sign, the word "contrast", "gadolinium" or "gad" on the scan within the small square. This indicates that contrast had been administered.

When reading scans you need to have a system and be methodical. A useful system is to approach the scan from the outside inward. Therefore, if we look at the large square of film that the scan is printed on, we start at the outside of the film and and look at the survey or scout image. This gives us a general idea of the way that the gantry of the scanner has been angled, by seeing the way that the lines go through the anatomical plane of the head and how many slices have been done. For instance, in the posterior fossa it is usual to do thinner cuts than in the rest of the brain. When presenting a scan you would start by saying "This is a contrasted (or uncontrasted) axial, sagittal or coronal CT/MRI (T1 or T2 weighted) scan of (person's name) done on (date of scan) and the most striking abnormality is ……"

Progressing from the outside of the slice inward, look firstly at the bone and, if you have a CT scan with bony windows, concentrate on these first. When looking at CT scans, be aware that there are several suture lines in the skull. The most obvious sutures are the lambdoid and the coronal suture. The coronal suture is seen about a third of the way back from the anterior part of the skull and the lambdoid suture is seen in the region of the posterior fossa cuts, see figure 7. MRI sequences are of little or no benefit when evaluating bone.

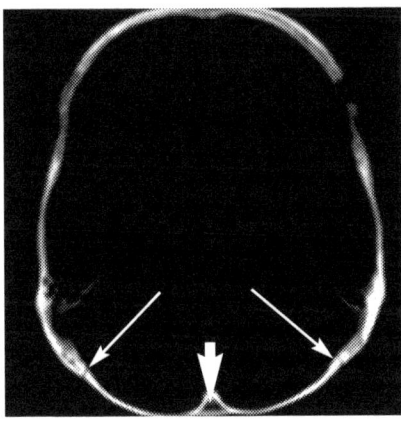

Figure 7. *This is a bone window of an axial CT scan. Both lambdoid sutures are indicated with the thin white arrows and the internal occipital protuberance with the thick white arrow. Note the burrhole in the left frontal region.*

Then, as far as the substance of the cerebrum is concerned, try to look for asymmetry. The sulcal pattern is a useful adjunct in this as a mass lesion in a hemisphere may flatten the sulcal pattern on that side. The sulci can be seen best on the convexity of the brain, at the top half, in the first few cuts from the vertex downward. When identifying lesions on a scan it is important to be able to describe them. You need to describe whether the lesion is homogenous or not. There might be a central necrotic or cystic component with the lesion having heterogeneous appearance of both solid tumour and cyst or it may be a homogenous (uniform density), solid tumour. Does the lesion have an irregular or regular outline, does it enhance with contrast and is there any associated oedema or mass effect? Having carefully studied the cerebral hemispheres, it is important to then focus on the ventricular system.

Hydrocephalus and ventriculomegaly

Any dilatation of the ventricular system or asymmetry should be noted. When the ventricles are dilated, it may be due to brain atrophy (hydrocephalus ex vacuo) and in this case the sulcal pattern will be enlarged as well as the basal cisterns. Alternatively, it could be due to hydrocephalus, in which case the ventricles become larger but the sulcal pattern and the basal cisterns become smaller due to the compressive effect of the ventricles. It is important to differentiate between communicating and non-communicating hydrocephalus. A basic rule is that if all four the ventricles are large then the ventricles are all communicating with each other and it is therefore communicating hydrocephalus. If there are one or two ventricles that are large and the rest are small then it is non-communicating hydrocephalus. For instance, a colloid cyst of the third ventricle will block off the foramina of Monroe and will cause both lateral ventricles to distend. The fourth ventricle which is not in communication with the lateral ventricles, due to an obstruction at the level of foramen of Monroe, will be normal in size, and this a non-communicating pattern of hydrocephalus. In communicating hydrocephalus, the obstruction is outside of the ventricular system and it can either be because the subarachnoid spaces and cisterns are obliterated, the outlet foramina are obstructed or because there is decreased absorption by the arachnoid villae.

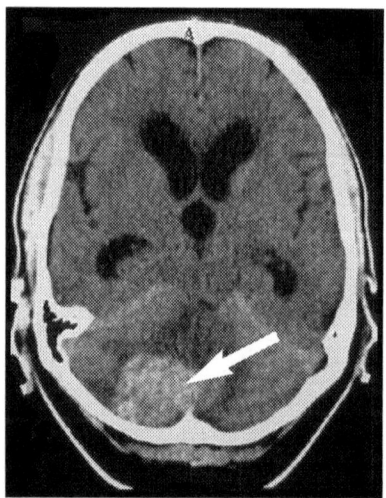

Figure 8. *Obstructive hydrocephalus. This is an uncontrasted axial CT scan. There is a haemorrhage in the posterior fossa (arrow) which is obstructing the fourth ventricle leading to obstructive hydrocephalus with dilatation of both anterior and temporal horns of the lateral ventricles and also dilatation of the third ventricle.*

When evaluating the posterior fossa, it is important to note that the vermis is usually of a different colour than the two cerebellar hemispheres. It can be easy to confuse the normal appearance of the vermis with that of a tumour. In patients presenting after a head injury it is important to evaluate the skull base for fractures. These are seen best on the bony cuts of the CT scan, which should be performed in all traumatic cases.

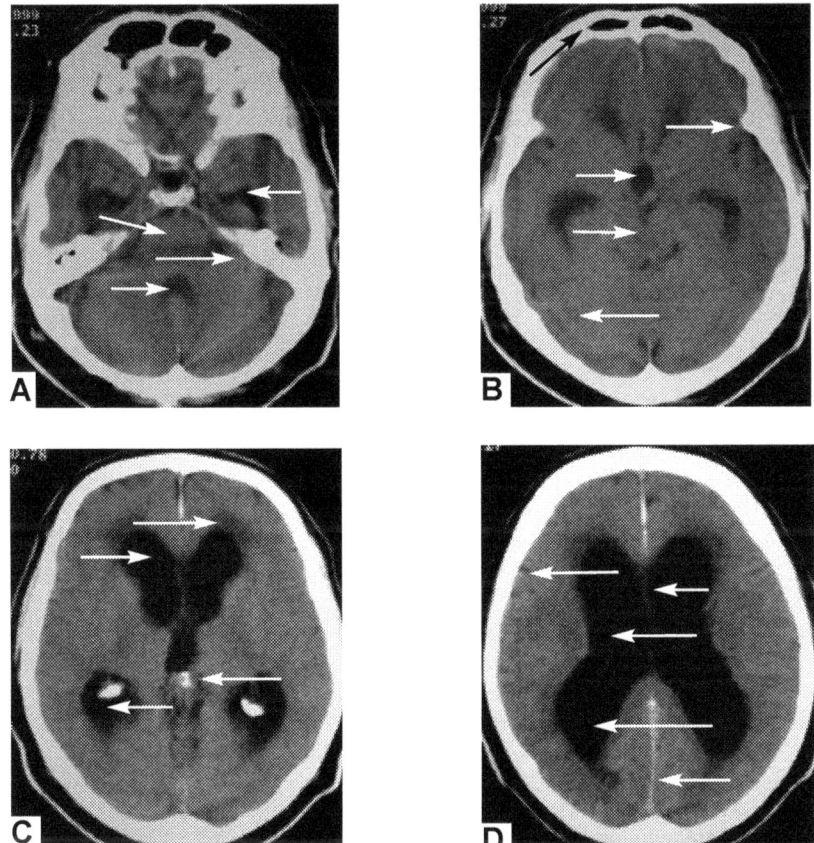

Figure 9. These are uncontrasted axial CT scans. In these images communicating hydrocephalus is depicted with dilatation of all the ventricles and the arrows are described from top to bottom; A: The top arrow demonstrates the dilated temporal horn of the left lateral ventricle, the next arrow demonstrates the pons, the next arrow demonstrates the left petrous part of the temporal bone and the last arrow shows the dilated fourth ventricle; B: The top arrow demonstrates the frontal air sinus, the next arrow the top part of the sphenoid ridge of the left temporal bone, next arrow demonstrates the dilated third ventricle, the next arrow the midbrain and the last arrow demonstrates the folia of the right cerebellar hemisphere; C: The top arrow demonstrates periventricular lucency due the increased hydrostatic pressure of CSF in the ventricle, the next arrow demonstrates the dilated frontal horn of the right lateral ventricle, the next arrow demonstrates the pineal gland and the next arrow the trigone of the right lateral ventricle containing choroid plexus; D: The top arrow depicts a cerebral sulcus, the next the septum pellucidum, the next demonstrates the body of the right lateral ventricle, the next the occipital horn of the right lateral ventricle and the last arrow demonstrates the falx cerebri.

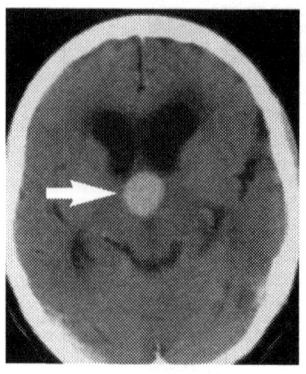

Figure 10. *Obstructive hydrocephalus. A colloid cyst of the third ventricle blocks both the foramina of Monroe bilaterally leading to obstructive hydrocephalus of the lateral ventricles.*

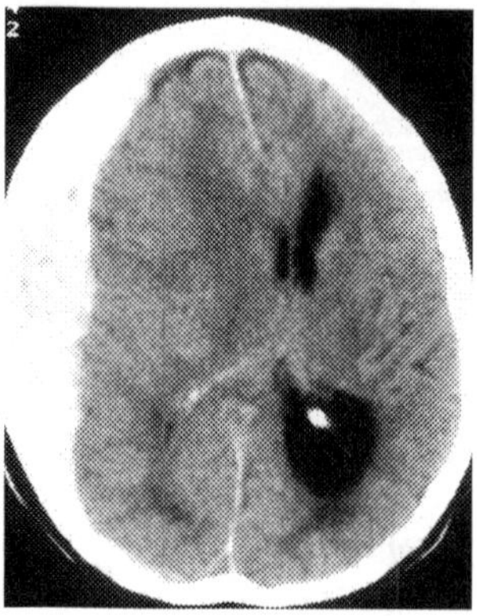

Figure 11. *Obstructive hydrocephalus. This is an uncontrasted axial CT scan. The acute subdural haemorrhage on the right has caused midline shift and trapped the frontal and occipital horns of the left lateral ventricle leading to dilatation and hydrocephalus.*

Trauma

A CT scan is the preferred investigation for cranial trauma. It does not require MR compatible ventilators or instruments, is simple, fast and widely available. The images are very sensitive for acute haemorrhage as well as cerebral oedema. CT scans are also the preferred imaging modality for evaluating bone and is an excellent tool for diagnosing fractures of the skull base, skull vault and facial bones. In trauma, the main categories of pathology are skull fractures, diffuse brain injury, intracerebral haemorrhages and extra-axial haemorrhages.

Skull fractures

The telltale sign of a skull fracture on a CT scan is usually overlying soft tissue swelling or disruption of the soft tissue with gas in the tissue. Fractures may be linear or depressed, comminuted or simple. Depressed fractures are frequently associated with dural tears and underlying intracerebral haemorrhages. Base of skull fractures may be difficult to identify, as they can often be hairline cracks. Fluid in the mastoid air cells or in the frontal sinus (opacification of the sinus) is frequently an indication of a skull base fracture with an associated dural tear and CSF leak. Intracranial air is another indication of a dural tear.

Diffuse brain injury

Diffuse brain injury (DBI) is part of a wide spectrum ranging from concussion to severe diffuse axonal injury. The hallmark of diffuse brain injury is pinpoint haemorrhage. These occur due to acceleration -deceleration and rotational forces imparted to the brain with subsequent tears in the white matter tracts, leading to pin point haemorrhages. They are usually found at the grey – white matter interface.

There are three grades of DBI:

Grade 1 – diffuse point bleeds throughout the brain.
Grade 2 – as above with point bleeds in the corpus callosum and
Grade 3 – as grade 2 with point bleeds in the dorsal mid-brain.

These 3 grades correlate well with prognosis and mid-brain haemorrhages are usually associated with a poor prognosis. Acute subdural haematomas are frequently associated with DBI as the rotational forces and acceleration - deceleration forces can lead to the draining veins suspended between the dura and the cortical surface being torn with subsequent haemorrhage into the subdural space.

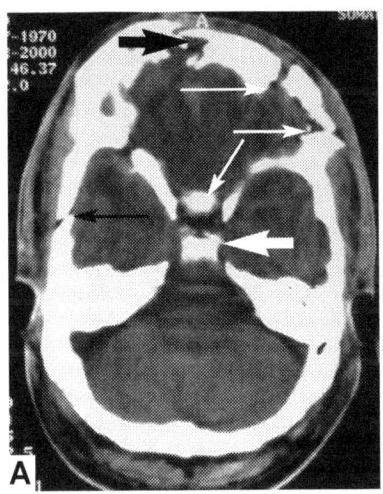 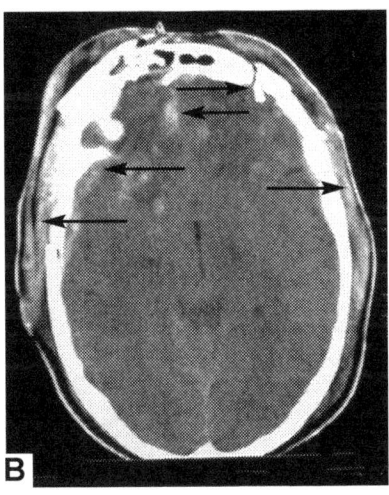

Figure 12. *These are uncontrasted axial CT scans. These images depict severe cranial trauma. A: The top 3 arrows depict a comminuted fracture of the frontal bone involving the frontal air sinus, the lower black arrow depicts a fracture of the right temporal bone, the angled arrow shows the tuberculum sellae and the thick white arrow the dorsum sellae B: The top arrow demonstrates a linear fracture of the frontal bone, the next demonstrates frontal lobe haemorrhagic contusions, the next a thin acute subdural haematoma and the last two arrows demonstrate extracranial soft tissue swelling secondary to traumatic impacts.*

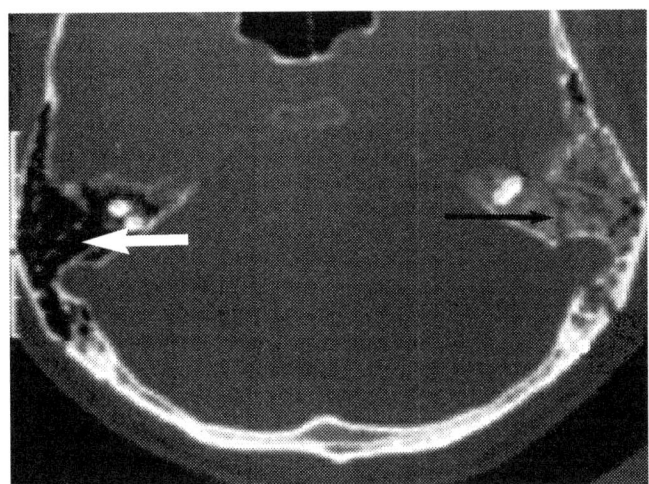

Figure 13. *This is the bone window of an axial CT scan. The black arrow depicts a transverse fracture of the petrous part of the temporal bone. This base of skull fracture has opacified the mastoid air cells on the left. The normal black appearance of the right sided mastoid air cells (thick arrow) is because they are filled with air whereas the white opacified air cells on the right are filled with fluid secondary to the fracture.*

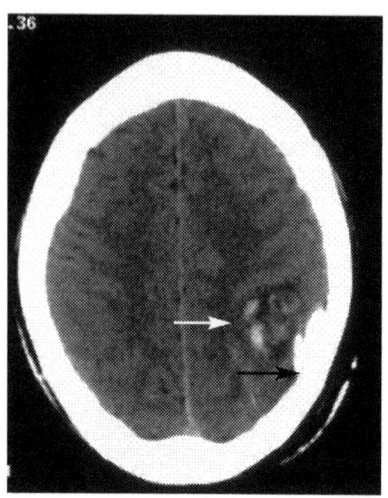 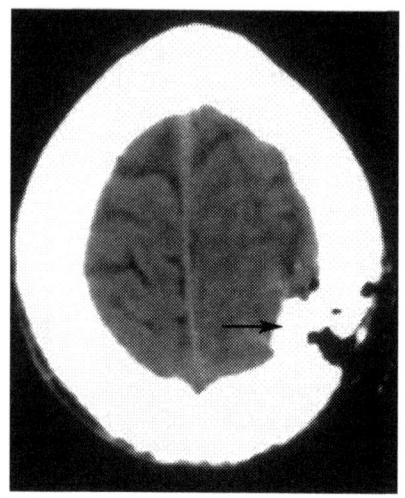

Figure 14. *These are uncontrasted axial CT scans. A comminuted, depressed fracture is depicted on these two axial slices (black arrows) with an underlying haemorrhagic contusion (white arrow). This is a typical example of focal brain trauma.*

Diffuse Injury Grade	CT appearance	Mortality
I	Normal CT scan	9.6%
II	Basal cisterns not effaced and midline shift < 5mm	13.5%
III	Cisterns compressed or absent and midline shift < 5mm	34%
IV	Shift > 5mm but no mass lesion of >25 cm^3 present	56.2%

Table 1. *The Marshall classification.*
(Marshall LF, Bowers-Marshall S, Klauber MR et al. A new classification of head injury based on computerised tomography. J Neurosurg 75 (Suppl):S14-20, 1991)

Intracerebral haemorrhage

We frequently see coup and contrecoup injuries where the impact side (coup side) as well as the opposite side (contrecoup side) demonstrates traumatic brain damage. This may for instance happen when a person falls onto the back of their head. The patient will have focal soft tissue swelling over the occiput with some focus of pathology there, frequently an intracerebral haemorrhage with some associated subarachnoid haemorrhage. Also the brain then moves forward and rubs over the rough surface of the orbital roof in the anterior cranial fossa and the frontal lobe poles impact against the inner skull leading to bifrontal contusions. There are frequently associated bitemporal contusions as the anterior poles of the temporal lobes collide with the sphenoid ridge, which forms the anterior border of the middle cranial fossa. These are devastating injuries and with longterm sequelae. These contusions quite often "blossom" as they enlarge and have associated oedema, usually about a week after the injury. Other intracerebral haemorrhages, called haemorrhagic contusions, can be larger versions of the pinpoint bleeds in diffuse brain injury and are caused by the same mechanism.

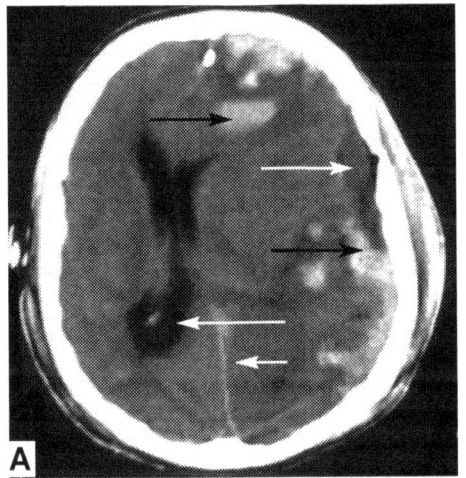 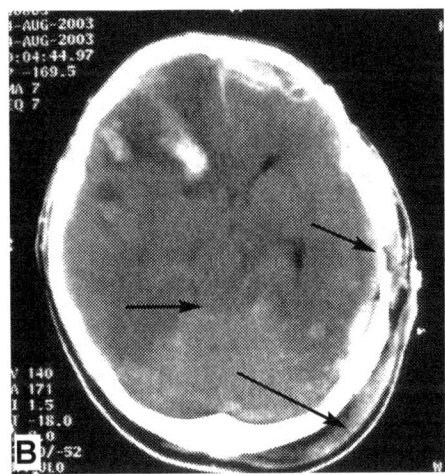

Figure 15. *These are uncontrasted axial CT scans. Both images depict severe diffuse brain injury. Note how on the left the hemisphere has swollen up and is herniating across the midline. A: The top arrow depicts a haemorrhagic contusion and several of these can be seen throughout both hemispheres, the next arrow demonstrates a hyperacute component of an acute subdural haematoma where the blood is so fresh that it has not yet had the time to clot and become hyperdense. It is important not to confuse this with a chronic subdural haematoma which has the same density. The next arrow demonstrates the clotted component of the acute subdural haematoma, the next arrow demonstrates the trapped ventricles due to midline shift and the last arrows demonstrates a parafalcine acute subdural haematoma. B: The top arrow shows a skull fracture. The next arrow demonstrates obliteration of the basal cisterns due to brain swelling. The last arrow demonstrates the widespread soft tissue swelling secondary to focal impacts. In this case the haemorrhagic contusions, acute subdural haematoma and parafalcine subdural haematoma point towards a diffuse brain injury with acceleration-deceleration and rotational forces and the skull fracture to a focal, impact type injury. This is typical for motor vehicle accidents where there is a combination of these mechanisms of injury.*

Extra-axial collections

Subdural and extradural collections may be difficult to tell apart. Subdural collections are usually craggy, irregularly shaped and depress the underlying brain. Epidural (extradural) haemorrhages are bicrescentic or biconvex lesions that strip the dura away from the bone. On CT scans both are white in the acute phase. In the hyperacute phase, before the blood has had a chance to clot, these lesions are darker than the brain and hypodense. Following the acute phase, the blood lyses and turns into deoxyhaemoglobin and bilirubin and it becomes more serous. The colour on CT scans changes to become more grey and eventually it becomes dark, very much the same density as the CSF. This happens over a couple of weeks. There is definite clinical significance in differentiating between a subdural and extradural haemorrhage. A subdural haemorrhage may sometimes continue to bleed but far more so, extradural haematomas have the propensity to do this. This gives rise to 'the talk and die' phenomenon where patients arrive in the hospital awake (the lucid interval) but then subsequently deterioratedue to ongoing haemorrhage from the ruptured vessel on the dural surface leading to increased haematoma formation and brain compression.

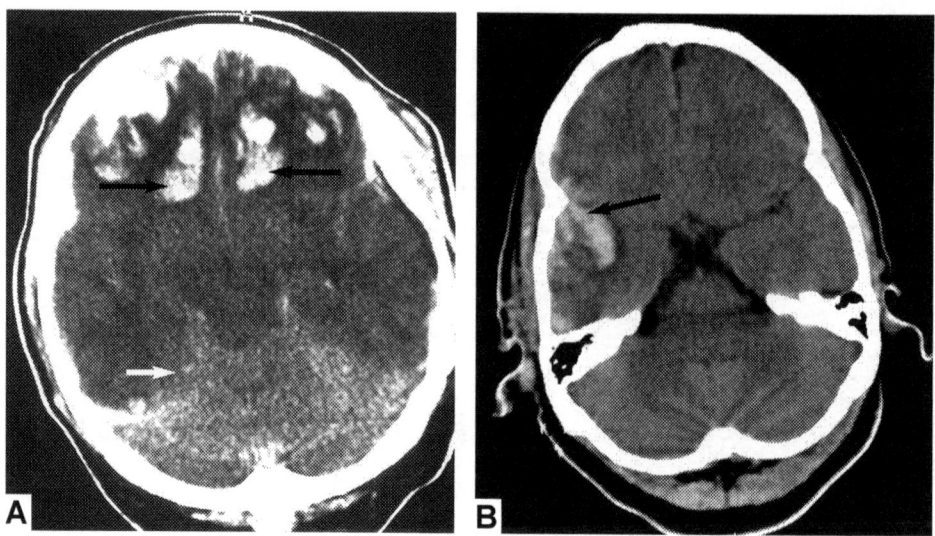

Figure 16. *These are uncontrasted axial CT scans. A: Note the severe bilateral haemorrhagic contusions (black arrows) and note the difference in density between the area of the tentorium cerebelli and the rest of the brain (white arrow). It can be difficult to tell whether this is due to ischaemia in the frontal and temporal lobes or is just the different imaging characteristics of the dura (tentorium cerebelli) and the brain parenchyma. These contusions are usually caused when the brain moves forward over the rough surface of the anterior cranial fossa; B: The movement of the brain cause the parenchyma of the frontal and temporal lobes adjacent to the Sylvian fissure to collide with the sphenoid ridge of the temporal bone, causing haemorrhagic contusions and in this case a small acute subdural haematoma (black arrow).*

When evaluating these lesions it is important to note their location, how big they are and what their effects are on the brain. When reporting these lesions, especially to a senior colleague, state the location of the haemorrhage and on how many cuts it can be seen on the CT scan as this indicates the total volume of the clot. CT scans are usually performed in 7 or 8mm cuts (the vertical distance between the slices) in the supratentorial area and therefore a haemorrhage that can be seen on 7 cuts is between 5-6cms high. When this is combined with the thickness of the clot you can get an estimate of how large it is. A haematoma 1 or 2 cm wide that can be seen on 4 or 5 cuts would be judged to be a large haematoma. It is sometimes difficult to visually separate the haematoma from the bone (since both are white) and if looking at the scans on the CT workstation it can be useful to change the settings of the scan (ask the radiographer to help you) and this frequently demonstrates the interface between the bone and the blood. Using Hounsfield units are also useful. It is important to look at the effect on the underlying brain and a midline shift of 5mm or more is significant. An extra-axial collection in the temporal lobe has much more clinical effect than a collection on the convexity as the temporal lobe is situated adjacent to the midbrain and even small haematomas can cause compression of the midbrain. It is easy to see the edge of the tentorium cerebelli at the medial border of the temporal lobe and it is possible to see herniation of the brain tissue (uncus) through this hiatus with subsequent compression of the brainstem. Acute extradural haematomas usually result from injury to the anterior or posterior branches of the middle meningeal artery. However, fractures associated with venous sinuses can also lead to extradural haematomas caused by a venous bleed rather than an arterial source. Venous extradural haematomas are more common in children. Subdural haematomas can also be interhemispheric or be found on the surface of the tentorium cerebelli.

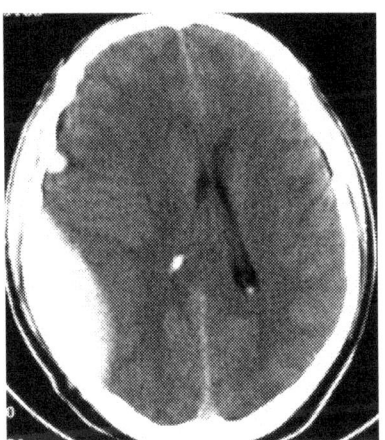

Figure 17. *This is an uncontrasted axial CT scan and it demonstrates an acute extradural haematoma with typical biconvex shape. This is because the dura is stripped away from the brain by the haematoma. These haematomas usually do not cross the suture lines.*

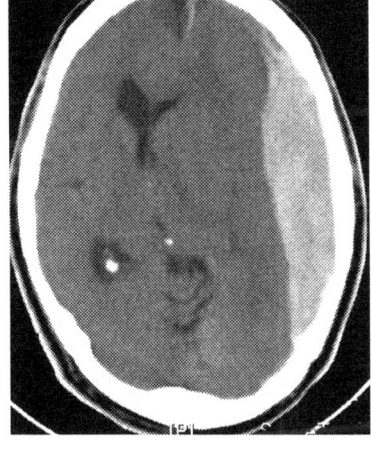

Figure 18. *This is an uncontrasted axial CT scan and it demonstrates an acute subdural collection with typical crescenteric shape. Note the marked midline shift as in figure 17 above.*

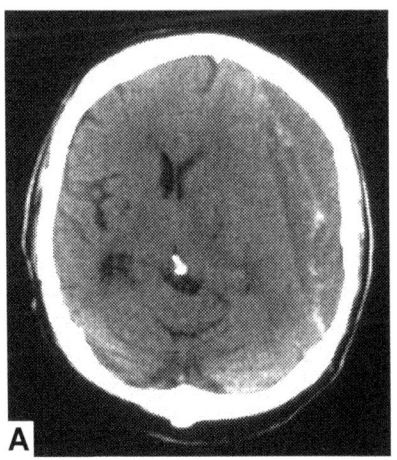

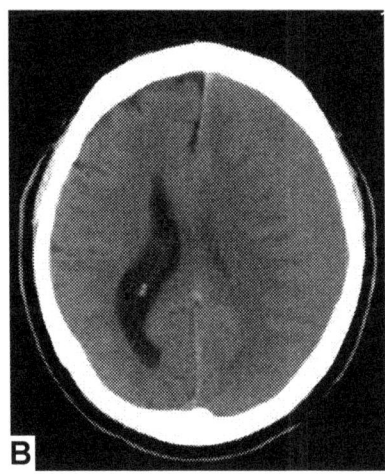

Figure 19. *These are uncontrasted axial CT scans. A: This chronic subdural haematoma is hypodense to brain. B: In this scan the subdural haematoma is isodense to brain making it very difficult to diagnose. It is the midline shift in these cases that make the diagnosis. The most difficult scenario is that of bilateral isodense subdural haematomas where there is no midline shift. In these cases, the ventricles will usually appear compressed and the basal cisterns and the sulci are also compressed.*

Brain tumours

Brain tumours can be either primary or secondary (metastasis). The administration of contrast medium greatly improves the CT sensitivity and specificity for tumour diagnosis. Enhancement with contrast may either represent blood-brain barrier breakdown or tumour neo-vascularity. Because of disruption of the normal cyto architecture in brain tumours, the blood-brain barrier does not remain intact and this allows seepage of contrast out of the vascular system. Similarly, the fast growing tissue of malignant tumours requires new blood vessels to feed the rapidly growing cells and this will lead to contrast enhancement at the area of the tumour. This is because tumours have more blood vessels and therefore more contrast density/intensity than the surrounding normal brain. Tumours are divided into intra-axial (within the neural axis that is the parenchyma of the brain or the spinal cord limited by the pia mater) and extra-axial tumours (outside of the neural axis and therefore outside the brain parenchyma and pia mater).

Primary brain tumours
(Low grade) astrocytoma
CT scan
Homogenous and frequently difficult to discern from brain
No contrast enhancement
Little surrounding oedema
MR scan
Homogenous and hypointense on T1 WI
Hyperintense on T2 WI
No contrast enhancement

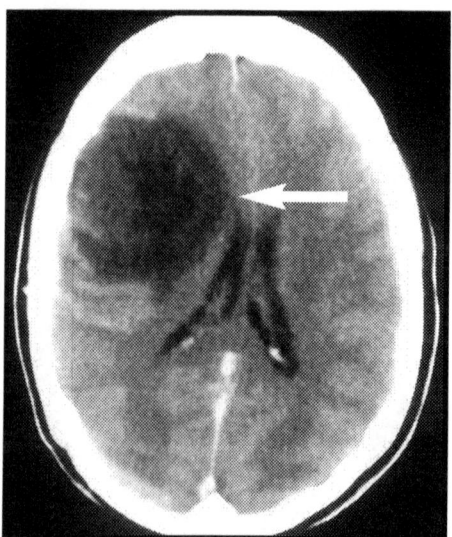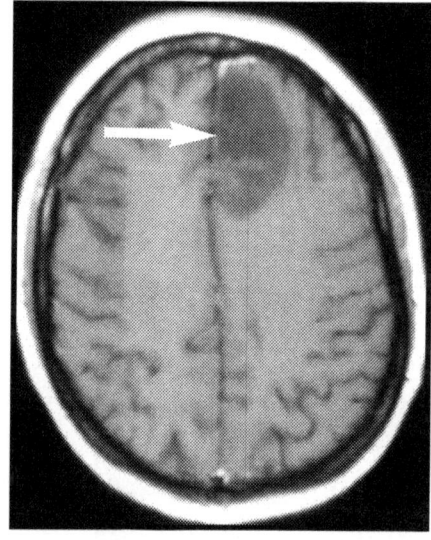

Figure 20. *The image on the left is a contrast enhanced axial CT scan and the image on the right is a contrast enhanced axial T1 WI. The hypodensities (arrows) on both scans are typical of low grade astrocytomas, as is the fact that they do not enhance.*

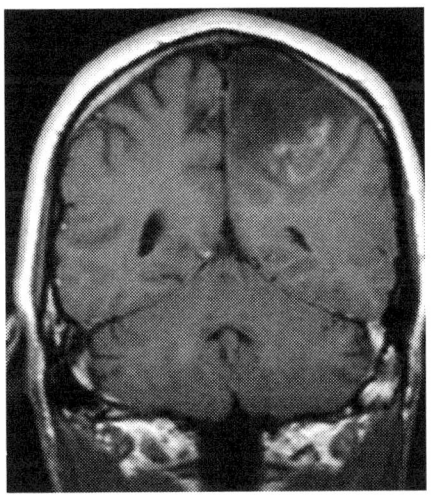 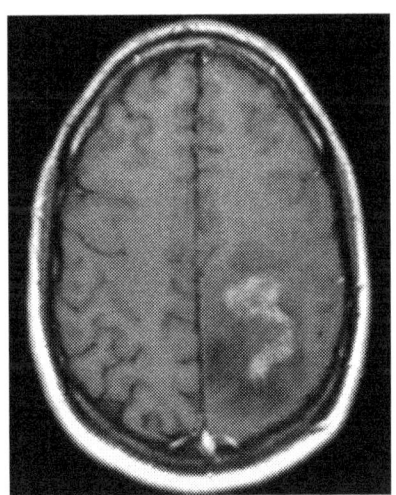

Figure 21. *Anaplastic astrocytoma. The scan on the left is a contrast enhanced coronal T1 WI and the scan on the right is a contrast enhanced axial T1 WI. The lesions are also hypodense on CT and hypointense on T1 WI like the low grade astrocytomas but, unlike the low grade astrocytomas, enhance with contrast.*

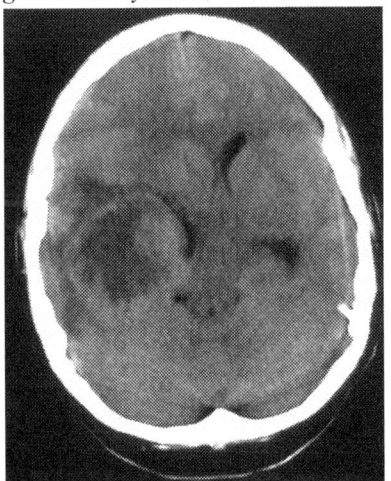 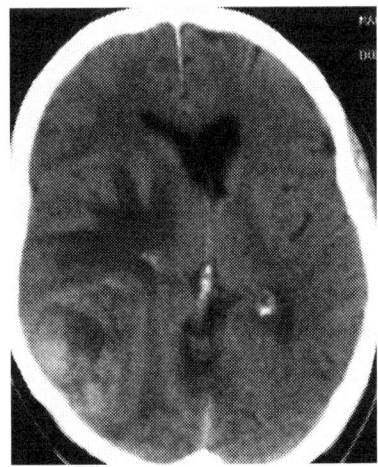

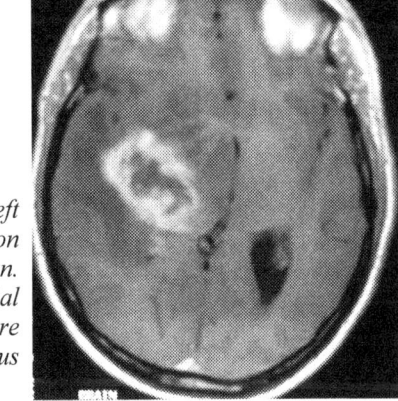

Figure 22. *Glioblastoma. The image on the top left is an uncontrasted axial CT scan and the image on the top right is a contrast enhanced axial CT scan. The image on the right is a contrast enhanced axial T1 WI. Glioblastomas have central necrosis, are irregular and craggy with strong heterogeneous enhancement and have surrounding oedema.*

Anaplastic astrocytoma
As for low grade astrocytoma but less homogenous, may have contrast enhancement

Glioblastoma Multiforme
CT scan
Heterogeneous with a hypodense centre
Strong but heterogeneous and irregular contrast enhancement
Surrounding oedema
Calcification indicates likely transformation from low grade.
MR scan
Heterogeneous and hypo/isointense on T1 WI
Hypointense centre on T1 WI (necrosis)
Strong and heterogeneous enhancement with contrast
Hyperintense on T2 WI
Surrounding oedema on T2 WI and FLAIR
The most important differential is that of an abscess which is usually round, thin walled and may be multiple

Pilocytic astrocytoma (mostly in children)
CT scan
Discrete solid or mixed solid/cystic mass found in the cerebral hemispheres or vermis
Hypo/iso dense to brain
No surrounding oedema
Calcified in 20%
Solid component enhances strongly
MR scan
Solid component hypo/isointense on T1 WI
Strong and heterogeneous enhancement with contrast
Solid component and cyst hyperintense on T2 WI, cyst does not suppress with FLAIR (abnormal fluid)

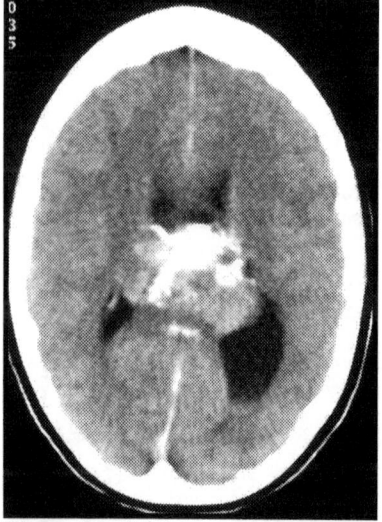

Figure 23. *Pilocytic astrocytoma. In this uncontrasted axial CT scan, this tumour has calcificied regions denoting a slow growth pattern These tumours are isodense or hypodense to brain and enhance strongly with contrast administration.*

Oligodendrogliomas (oligodendrocytes and glial cells)
CT scan
Hypo/isodense
Most are calcified
Variable enhancement
MR scan
Hypo/isointense on T1 WI
Half enhance with contrast.
Hyperintense on T2 WI

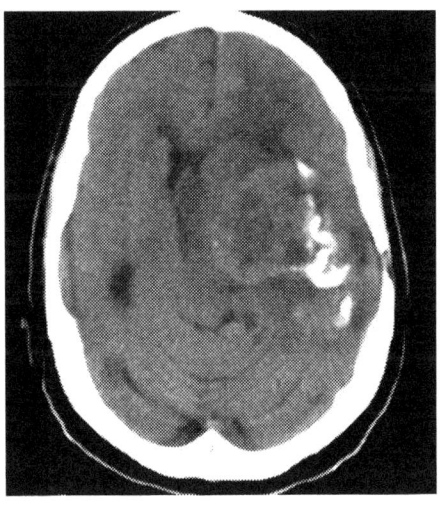

Figure 24. *Oligodendroglioma. In this uncontrasted axial CT scan, this tumour demonstrates calcification and is isodense to brain. In this case there was minimal contrast enhancement.*

Ependymoma
Posterior fossa (small children)
CT scan
Floor of fourth ventricle and cerebello-pontine angle
Isodense to brain
Half are calcified
Variable enhancement
Hydrocephalus
MR scan
Hypointense on T1 WI
Half enhance with contrast.
Isointense on T2 WI
Variable enhancement
Hydrocephalus

Supratentorial (older children and adults)
CT scan
Parenchymal or intraventricular mass
Heterogenous
Half are calcified
Hydrocephalus (in intraventricular tumours)
Variable enhancement
MR scan
Hypointense on T1 WI
Isointense on T2 WI
Variable enhancement
Hydrocephalus (in intraventricular tumours)

Meningiomas
CT scan
Mostly hyperdense
Calcification in 25%
Strong, homogenous enhancement
Associated bony changes such as osseous hypertrophy
MR scan

Isointense or slightly hyper intense on T1 WI
Isointense on T2 WI, surrounding oedema in half with decreased signal intensity on T2 if there is calcification.
Strong, homogenous enhancement, dural tail (origin from dura can be seen)

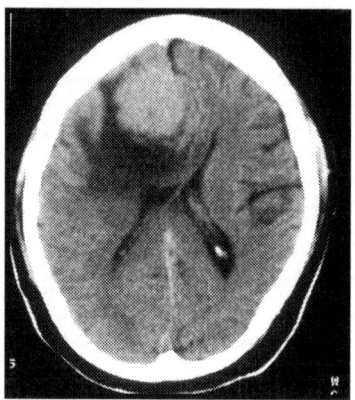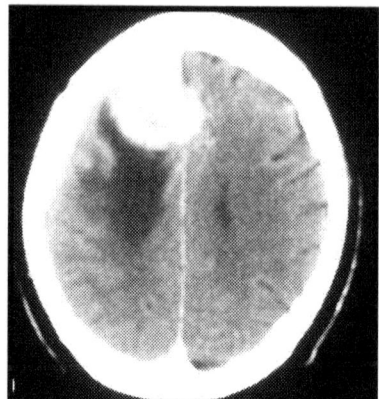

Figure 25. *Meningioma. The scan on the left is an uncontrasted axial CT scan of the brain and the scan on the right a contrast enhanced axial CT scan. The meningioma clearly demonstrates attachment to the dura of the falx, has a lot of surrounding oedema and enhances brilliantly with contrast.*

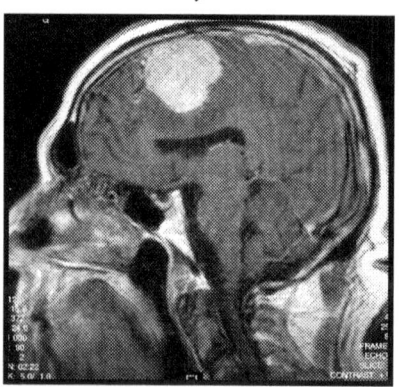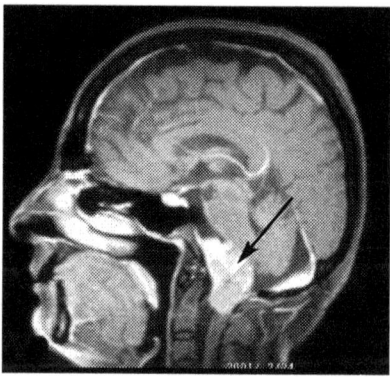

Figure 26. *The image on the left is a sagittal T1 WI following contrast administration. This also clearly demonstrates a dural attachment and brilliant contrast enhancement of the same meningioma as seen above. The image on the right is a contrast enhanced saggital T1WI scan and demonstrates a skull base meningioma occupying a large part of the foramen magnum (arrow).*

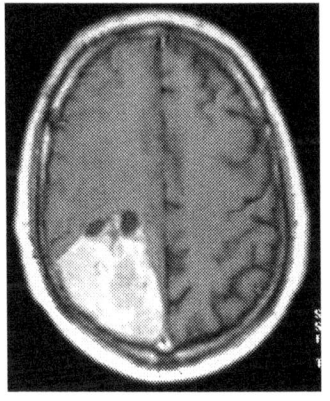 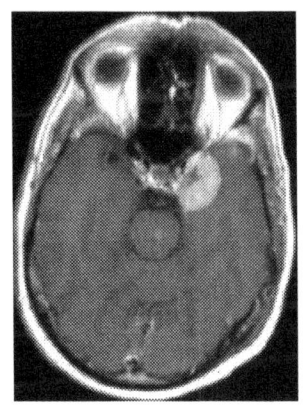

Figure 27. *The image on the left is a contrast enhanced axial T1 WI of the brain, demonstrating dural attachment and vivid enhancement of this convexity meningioma. The image on the right is a contrast enhanced axial T1 WI which clearly shows a meningioma of the left cavernous sinus.*

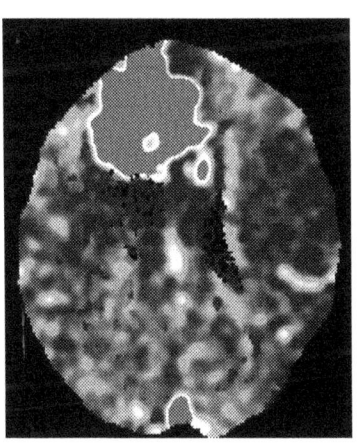

Figure 28. *This image demonstrates a dynamic perfusion CT scan which is performed using pixel density and transit time to measure flow and volume. It clearly demonstrates high flow and high blood volume within the same tumour as seen in figure 25.*

Primary central nervous system lymphoma
CT scan
Mostly hyperdense
Frequently in periventricular location
Moderate, homogenous enhancement
MR scan
Isointense on T1 WI
Isointense on T2 WI (hyperintense on FLAIR)
Strong, homogenous enhancement

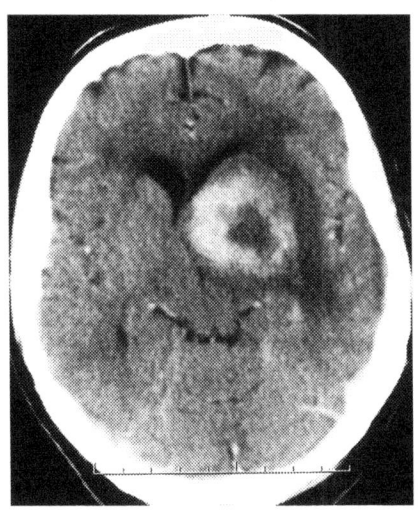

Figure 29. *Lymphoma. This uncontrasted axial CT scan demonstrates a high density periventricular lesion. Note the central area of necrosis and associated oedema.*

Intracranial cyst-like lesions
Dermoid cyst (located in midline)
CT scan
Hypodense (density of fat)
Does not enhance
MR scan
Hyperintense on T1 WI (hypointense on STIR)
Heterogenous on T2 WI
No enhancement
Epidermoid cyst (located in midline and cerebello-pontine angle)
CT scan
Hypodense (density of CSF)
May have some calcification
Does not enhance
MR scan
Hypointense on T1 WI
Hyperintense on T2 WI
Does not suppress on FLAIR sequence
No enhancement

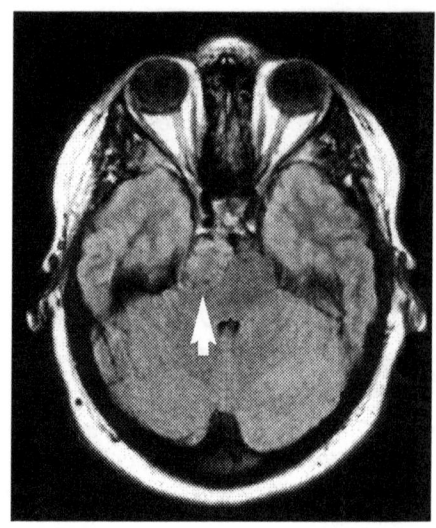

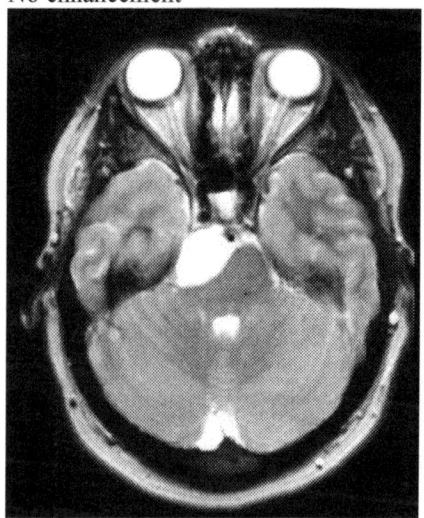

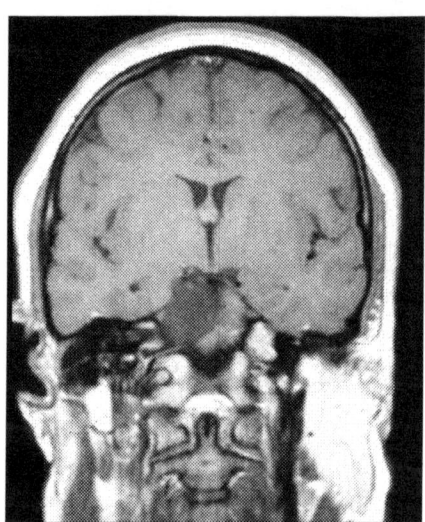

Figure 30. *The image on the left is an axial T2 WI and demonstrates an epidermoid cyst in the right cerebellopontine angle. Note that it is brightly intense on this image. A FLAIR image will have a similar intensity. The image on the top right is a T1 WI axial scan and the image on the bottom right is a coronal T1 WI. Note that the same lesion is hypointense on these images. It would not enhance on contrast enhanced images.*

Colloid cyst of the third ventricle
CT scan
Mostly hyperdense, can be isodense
Obstructive hydrocephalus
Does not enhance
MR scan
Variable on T1 WI and T2 WI
Does not enhance

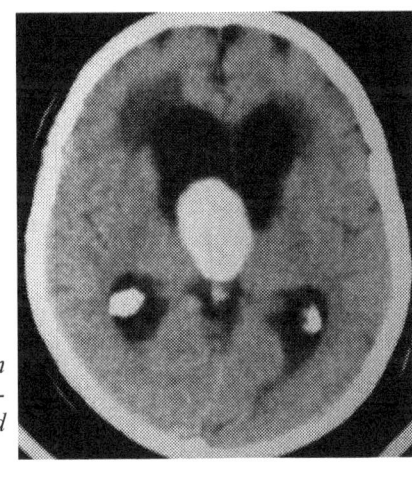

Figure 31. *Colloid cyst. This image is of an uncontrasted axial CT scan of the brain demonstrating a typical hyperdense lesion in the third ventricle with obstructive hydrocephalus.*

Arachnoid cysts (Sylvian fissure, basal cisterns, CPA)
CT scan
Mostly CSF density
Obstructive hydrocephalus
Does not enhance
MR scan
Same intensities as CSF
Does not enhance
Suppresses with FLAIR (used to discern from epidermoid cysts which do not suppress)

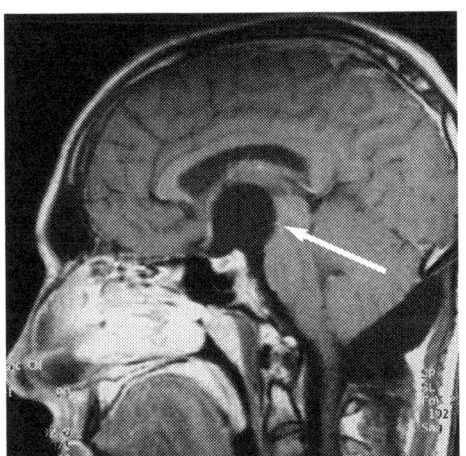 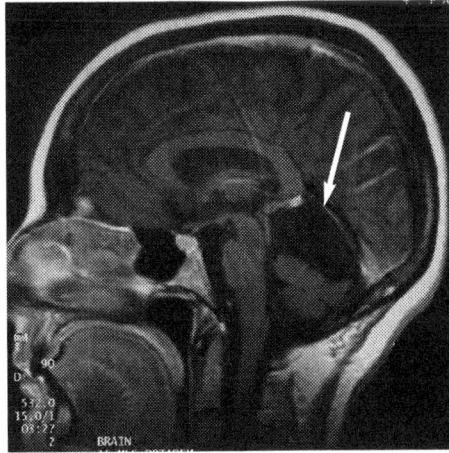

Figure 32. *These are uncontrasted sagittal T1 WI scans. The scan on the left demonstrates a suprasellar arachnoid cyst. the image on the left demonstrates an arachnoid cyst in the posterior fossa.*

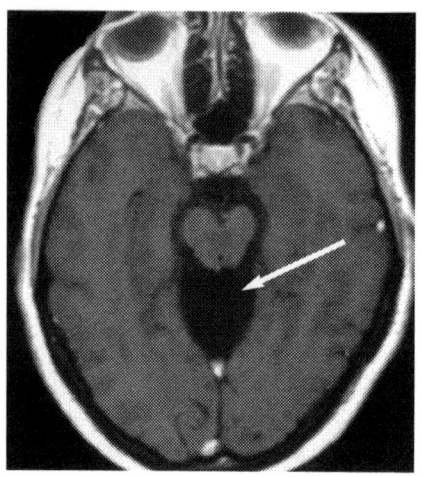

Figure 32a. *This image is an axial T1 WI demonstrating an arachnoid cyst of the posterior fossa. Note the CSF density of the lesion.*

Pituitary region tumours
Microadenomas (<1cm)
CT scan
Not seen, may be seen following contrast
MR scan
Variable on T1 WI and T2 WI
May enhance

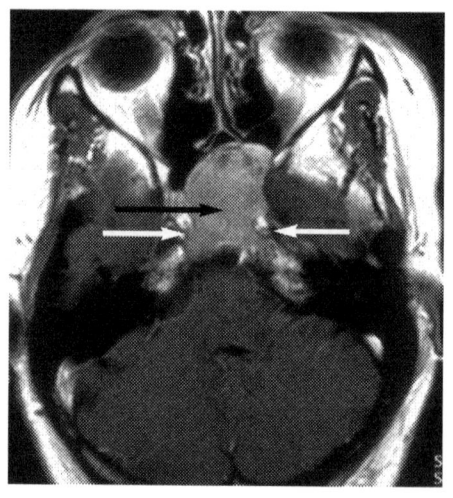

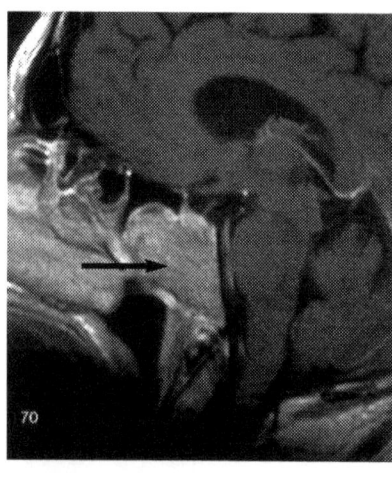

Figure 33. *The image on the left is a sagittal contrast enhanced T1 WI and the image above is an axial contrast enhanced T1 WI. Both show a pituitary macroadenoma (black arrows) with the axial image showing involvement of the cavernous sinuses bilaterally (white arrows).*

Macroadenomas (>1cm)
CT scan
Mostly isodense
Cysts/necrosis common
Usually enhances
May show signs of erosion and have extra sellar extension
MR scan
Isointense to gray matter on T1 WI and T2 WI
Usually enhances
Extra sellar extension may occur
Always look for haemorrhage

Craniopharyngiomas

CT scan
Mostly cystic
Calcified
Enhances

MR scan
Variable on T1 WI and T2 WI
Tend to erode the posterior clinoid
Hydrocephalus

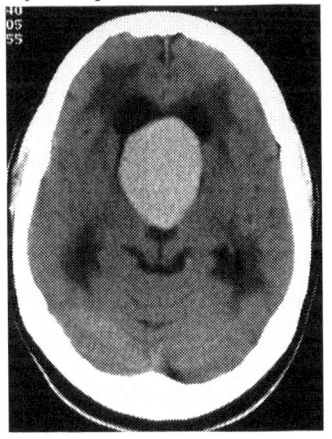 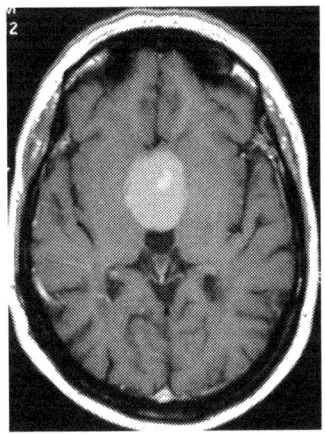

Figure 34. *The image on the left is a contrast enhanced axial CT scan and the image on the right is an unenhanced axial T1 WI. The craniopharyngioma enhances with contrast on the CT scan and is naturally hyperintense on the T1 WI because of the high lipid content of the tumour.*

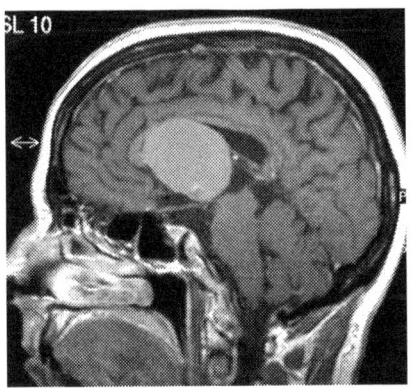 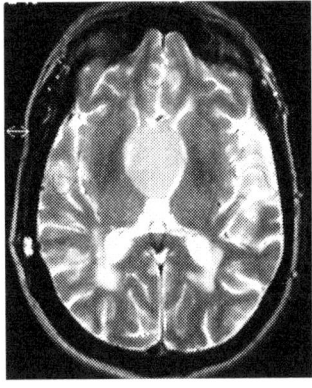

Figure 35. *The image on the left is an unenhaced sagittal T1 WI and the image on the right is a T2 WI axial scan of the brain. Note how the craniopharyngioma is hyperintense on both due to its high lipid (T1 WI) and fluid content (T2 WI)*

Neuronal tumours
Central neurocytomas (intraventricular)

CT scan
Mixed solid/cystic
Heterogeneous
Calcified in 50%

Enhances heterogeneously
MR scan
Isointense T1 WI
Hyperintense T2 WI
Inhomogeneous
Enhances heterogeneously
Hydrocephalus

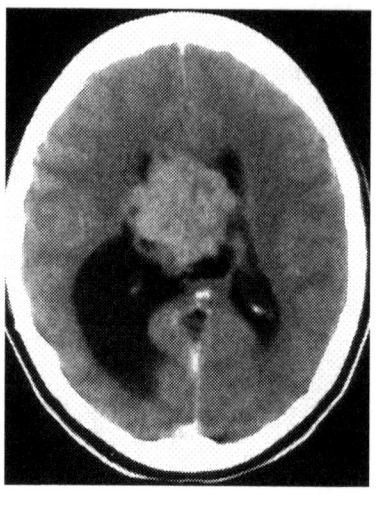

Figure 36. *This unenhanced axial CT scan of the brain demonstrates a central neurocytoma. These lesions are frequently heavily calcified and enhance with contrast and are histologically similar to oligodendrogliomas.*

Pineal region tumours
Germinoma (lesion infiltrates and displaces the pineal gland)
CT scan
Iso/hyperdense lesion at the posterior aspect third ventricle (pineal region)
Hydrocephalus
Enhances strongly
MR scan
Iso/hypointense T1 WI
Hyperintense T2 WI
Inhomogeneous
Enhances strongly and heterogeneously

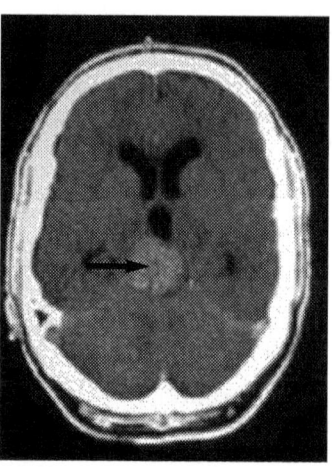

Figure 37. *Germinoma. This is an unenhanced axial CT scan. Tumours of the pineal region can be very difficult to tell apart as they all share some features. However, this lesion demonstrates infiltration and destruction of the pineal which is typical for germinomas.*

Pineal parenchymal tumours (lesion grows from inside out, displacing pineal circumferentially)
Pinealocytoma
CT scan
Iso/hypodense posterior aspect third ventricle (pineal region)
Does not enhance
Hydrocephalus
MR scan
Iso/hypointense T1 WI
Hyperintense T2 WI
Well delineated
Enhances strongly

Pinealoblastoma
CT scan
Heterogeneous lesion
Enhances heterogeneously
Hydrocephalus
MR scan
Iso/hypointense T1 WI
Hyperintense T2 WI
Poorly delineated
Enhances strongly
Demonstrates local infiltration

Tumours of the posterior fossa
Hemangioblastoma (Association with Von Hippel-Lindau disease)
CT scan
Low density cyst
Enhancing mural nodule
Sometimes solid enhancing tumour
MR scan
Iso/hypointense T1 WI
Hyperintense T2 WI
Nodule enhances strongly

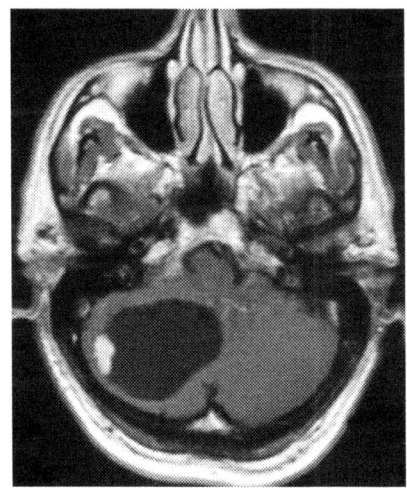

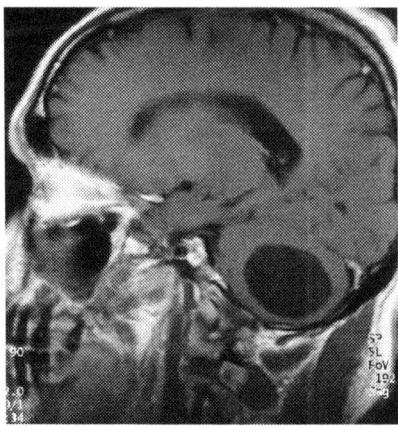

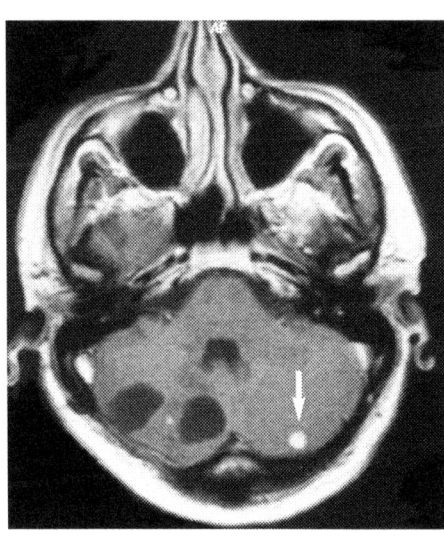

Figure 38. *These are contrast enhanced T1 WI. The top image is a T1 WI demonstrating the classical appearance of a hemangioblastoma. Note the large cyst with an enhancing mural nodule. The bottom right image is a sagittal scan of the same lesion. The image on the left is an axial contrast enhanced T1 WI from a different patient and demonstrates multiple hemangioblastomas. There is also a nodule in the left cerebellum without an associated cyst (arrow).*

Medulloblastoma (Primitive neuro-ectodermal tumour of post fossa)
CT scan
Hyperdense, solid
Midline posterior fossa
Associated hydrocephalus common
Enhances fairly uniformly
MR scan
Midline homogenous posterior fossa tumour

Iso/hypointense T1 WI
Isointense T2 WI
Enhances
Drop metastasis (seeding through CSF)

Astrocytoma (see glial tumours)

Skull base tumours
Chordoma
CT scan
Hypodense mixed cystic and solid
Midline location
Commonly calcified
Bony destruction
Enhances heterogeneously
MR scan
Iso/hypointense T1 WI
Isointense T2 WI
Enhances heterogeneously

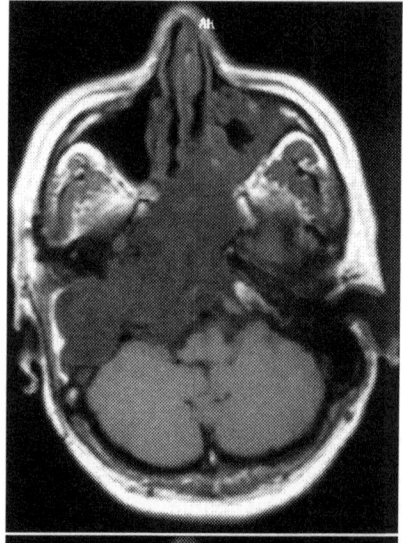

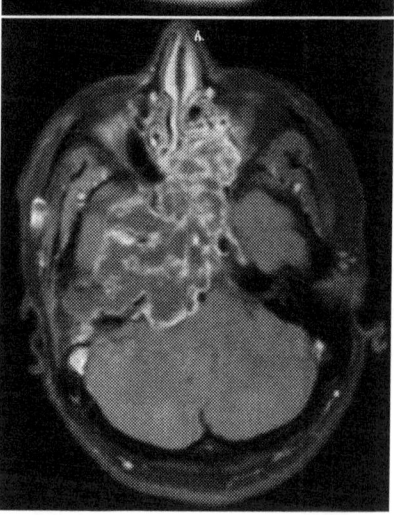

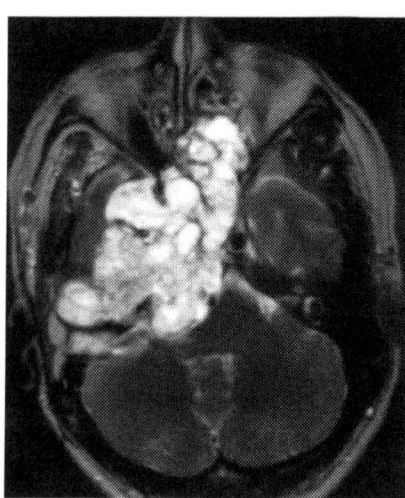

Figure 39. *The image on the top is an unenhanced axial T1 WI and the image on the bottom is a contrast enhanced T1 WI demonstrating an extensive skull base chordoma. Note the strong but inhomogeneous enhancement of the tumour.*

Figure 40. *This image is an axial T2 WI of the same patient and the high signal (and the low signal on the T1 WI) indicates the high fluid content of these tumours. The images demonstrate the highly aggressive infiltrative nature of these tumours.*

Vestibular Schwannoma
CT scan
Iso/hyperdense tumour in the cerebello-pontine angle
Solid or solid/cystic
Expanded internal auditory meatus

60

Enhances uniformly
MR scan
Iso/hypointense T1 WI
Hyperintense T2 WI
May be heterogenous/cystic components
Enhances strongly
Has a clear relation to the facial nerve on high-resolution scans

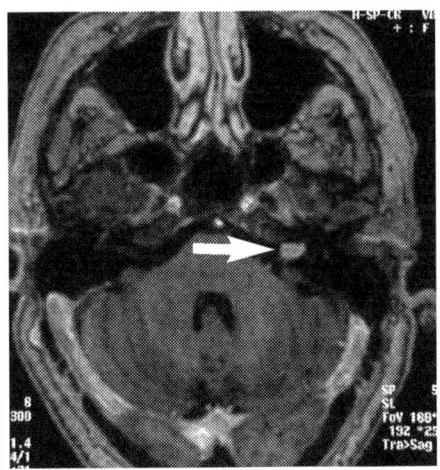

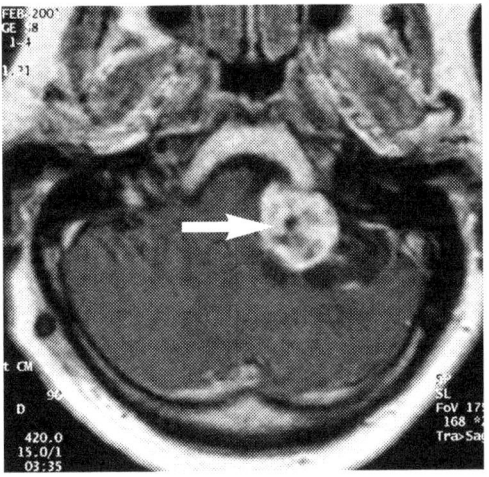

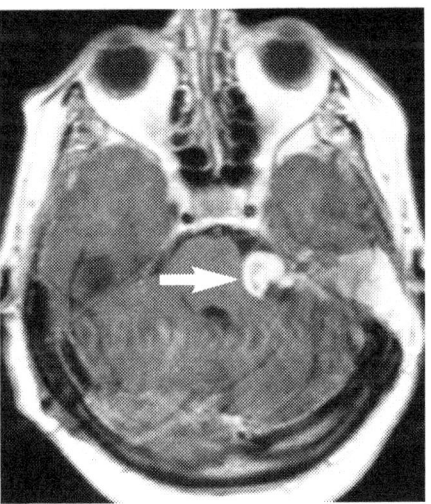

Figure 41. *These axial contrast enhanced T1 WI demonstrate different sizes of left sided vestibular schwannomas. The image top right demonstrates an intracanalicular schwannoma (white arrow). The image on the left demonstrates frank brainstem compression.*

Metastatic tumours
CT scan
Iso/hypodense tumour in parenchyma/dura
Severe surrounding oedema
Enhances strongly, frequently ring enhancing
MR scan
Iso/hypointense T1 WI
Hyperintense T2 WI
May have heterogeneous/cystic components
Enhances strongly
Severe surrounding oedema

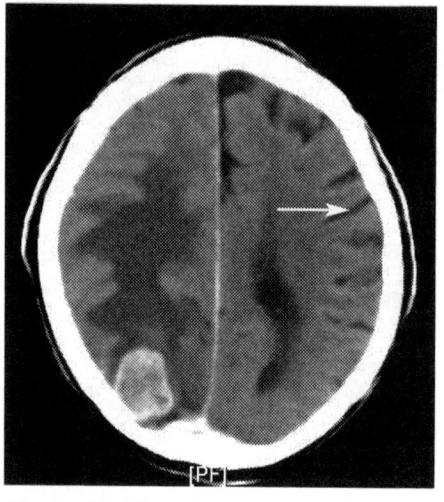 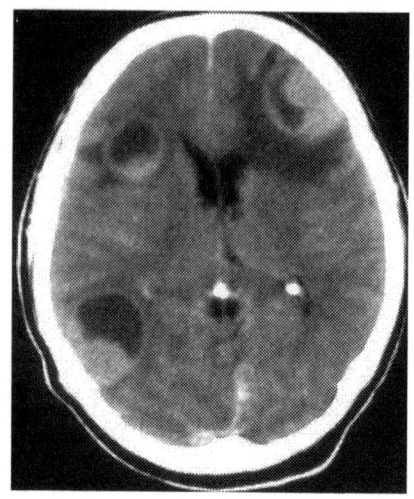

Figure 42. *These images are contrast enhanced axial CT scans of the brain. The image on the left demonstrates a single metastasis in the right occipital lobe with surrounding brain oedema and effacement of the sulcal pattern. See the normal sulci in the left hemisphere (arrow). The image on the right demonstrates multiple metastases with surrounding oedema.*

Vascular Pathology
Arterial infarct
CT scan
May see hyperdense vessel (thrombosis)
Hypodensity after 24 hrs
Can be seen within hours on perfusion CT scan
May have haemorrhagic transformation after 24-48 hours
MR scan
Loss of grey white differentiation on T1 WI
Hyperintense T2 WI
Enhances with contrast

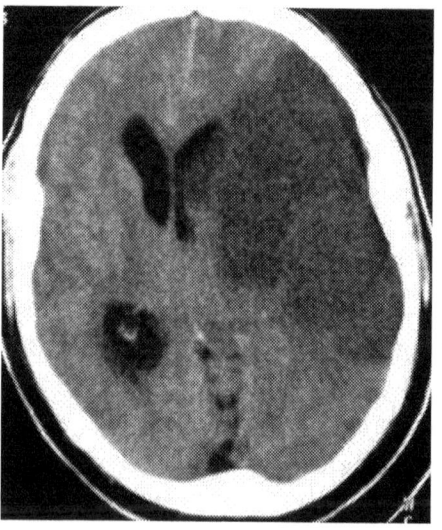

Figure 43. *This uncontrasted axial CT scan of the brain demonstrates an ischaemic infarct of the dominant left hemisphere in the middle cerebral artery distribution*

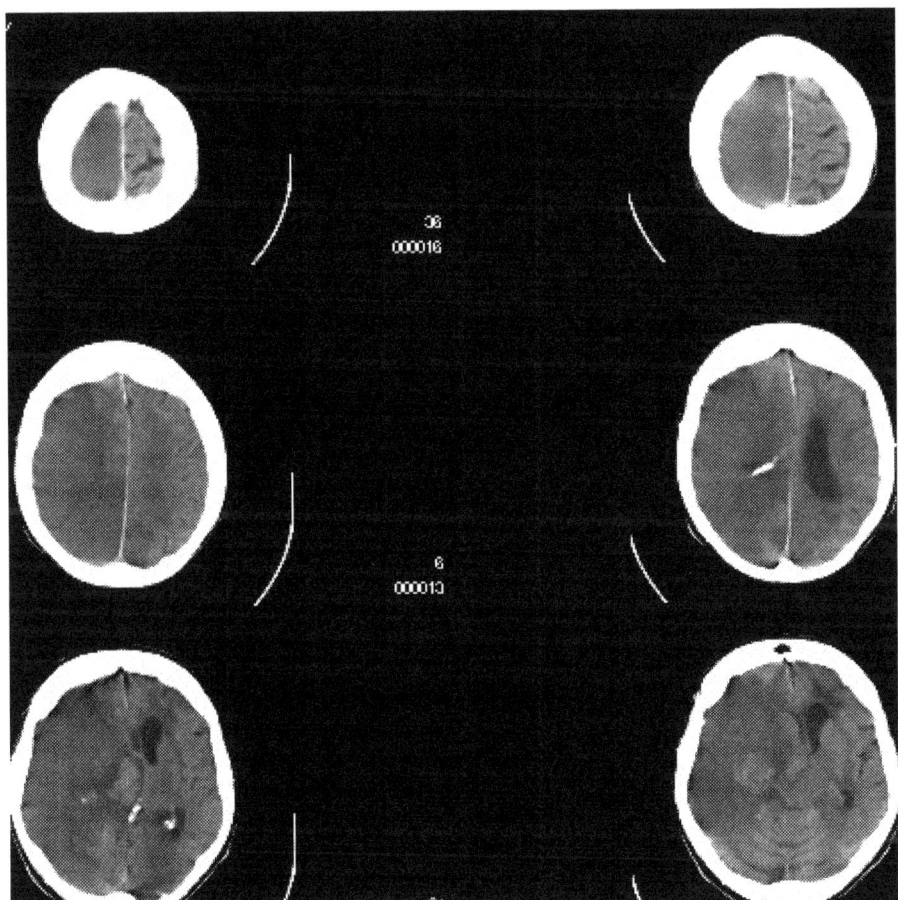

Figure 44. *This sequence of slices of an uncontrasted axial CT scan of the brain demonstrate an ischaemic infarct of the right, non dominant hemisphere in the distribution of the middle cerebral artery.*

Venous infarct
CT scan
Hyperdense sagittal sinus
Parenchymal petechial haemorrhages
Empty delta sign with contrast administration (enhancing dura around haematoma in confluence of sinuses)
MR scan
Haematoma seen in sinus
T1 WI in the acute stage isointense with brain, in the subacute stage hyperintense
Parenchymal swelling and haemorrhage, hyperintense on T2 WI

Spontaneous Haemorrhage
SAH (aneurysmal)
CT scan
Positive in 97% within 12 hours of haemorrhage and decreases to about 70% sensitivity on day 3.
Hyperdensity in basal cisterns and subarachnoid spaces.
Hydrocephalus (early hydrocephalus = dilated temporal horns, plump third ventricle)

Blood in occipital horns of lateral ventricles
May have subtle obliteration of Sylvian fissure
MR scan
Isointense with brain on T1 WI in the acute phase and hyperintense on T2 WI
Siderosis in the chronic phase is hypointense on T2 WI

Grade	Description
Fisher 0	Unruptured aneurysm
Fisher 1	No blood seen
Fisher 2	Diffuse blood and no vertical layers of blood > 1mm
Fisher 3	Clot and vertical layers of blood > 1mm
Fisher 4	Intracerebral haematoma or/and intraventricular blood

TABLE 2. *Fisher grading scale. This CT scan scale is used in SAH to predict vasospasm. The incidence of vasospasm is higher in Fisher 3 than 2, but lower in Fisher 4.*

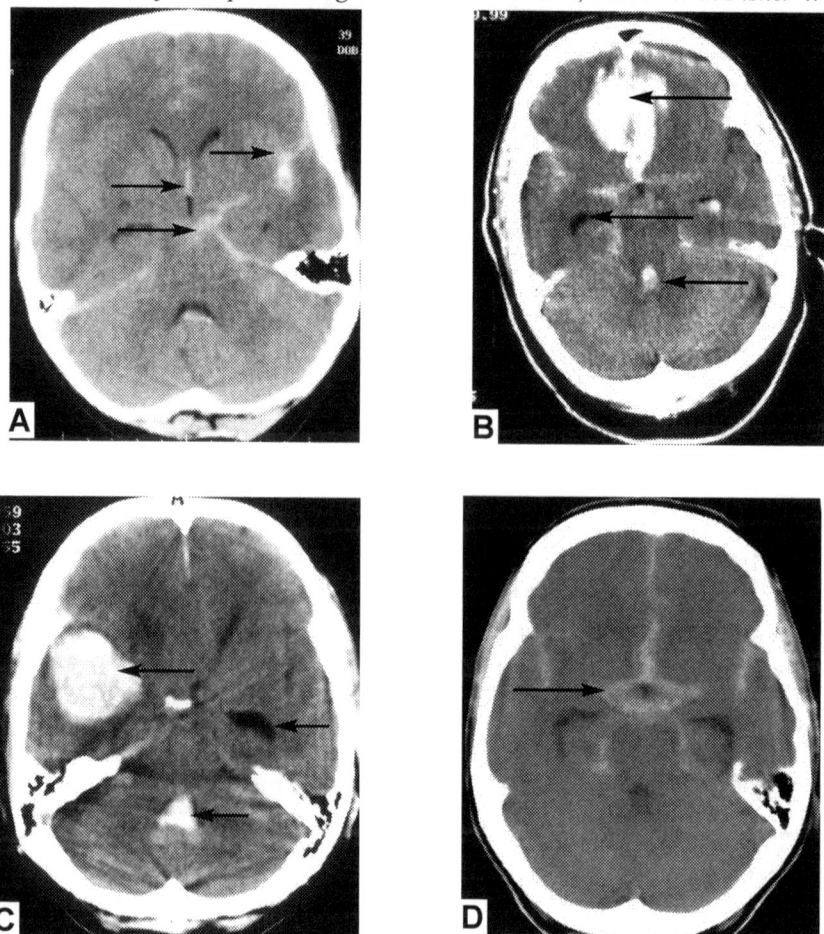

Figure 45. *See legend on opposite page.*

Figure 45. *(see opposite page) These images are uncontrasted axial CT scans demonstrating subarachnoid blood; A: The top arrow demonstrates fresh blood in the left Sylvian fissure, the next arrow demonstrates blood in the third ventricle and the last arrow demonstrates blood in the pre pontine cistern at the base of the brain;. B: The top arrow demonstrates an intraparenchymal haemorrhage secondary to an anterior communicating artery aneurysm. This is a pattern of blood indicative of this type of aneurysm. The next arrow demonstrates the dilated temporal horn of the right lateral ventricle and the last arrow demonstrates blood in the fourth ventricle; C: The top arrow demonstrates an intraparenchymal haemorrhage in the right Sylvian fissure, the next arrow demonstrates a dilated temporal horn and the last arrow, blood in the fourth ventricle; D: This image demonstrates the star shaped haemorrhage in the basal cisterns and the interhemispheric and Sylvian fissures that is classically associated with SAH.*

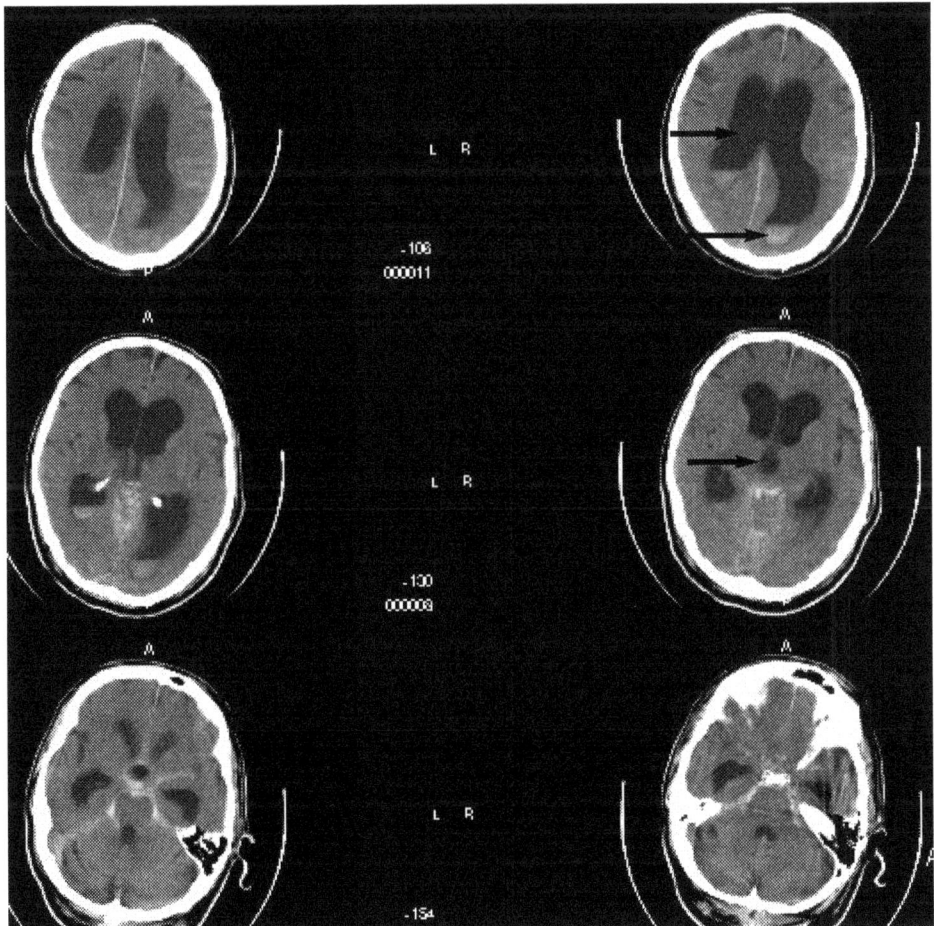

Figure 46. *This sequence of images are a selection from an uncontrasted axial CT scan demonstrating SAH. Notice how the classic star shape subarachnoid distribution of blood is seen in this sequence, also the associated hydrocephalus (top arrow) and blood in the ventricular system (second arrow). The whole of the ventricular system is dilated with the lateral ventricles, the third ventricle (bottom arrow) and the fourth ventricle dilated, indicating communicating hydrocephalus.*

Parenchymal hypertensive haemorrhage
CT scan
Hyperdense mass (clotted blood)
Seen in several sites including putamen, insula, brainstem, posterior fossa
MR scan
Depends on age of clot
In T1 WI – remember 'Big Great White Bear!'
Hyperacute, within hours - **B**lack (hypointense)
Acute stage, less than 3 days - **G**rey (isointense),
Subacute stage, 3 to 14 days - **W**hite (hyperintense),
Chronic stage, more than 14 days - **B**lack (hypointense)

In T2 WI – remember 'Bear, What Bear?'
Acute stage – **B**lack (hypointense)
Subacute – **W**hite (hyperintense)
Subacute stage and chronic stages – **B**lack (hypointense)

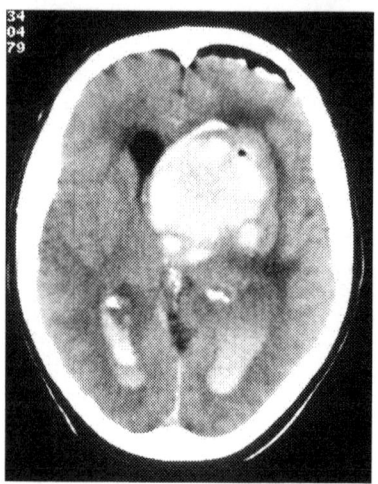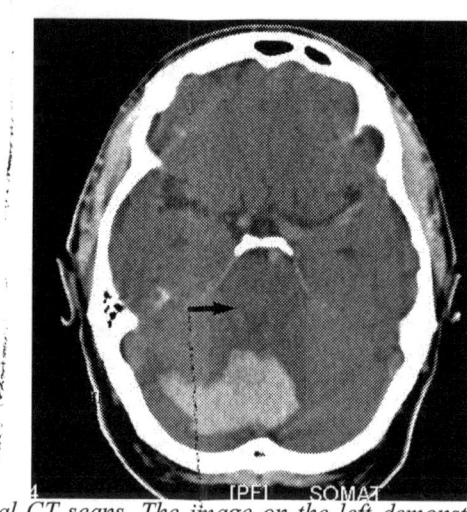

Figure 47. *These are uncontrasted axial CT scans. The image on the left demonstrates a spontaneous parenchymal intracerebral haemorrhage in the region of the left basal ganglia and internal capsule with extension into the ventricular system. The image on the right demonstrates a posterior fossa spontaneous intraparenchymal intracerebellar haemorrhage with compression and occlusion of the basal cisterns (arrow) and fourth ventricle.*

Vascular anomalies
AVM (arteriovenous malformation)
CT scan
Hyperdense serpentine vessels
Enhances strongly with contrast
MR scan
Flow voids on T1 WI, enhances strongly with contrast
Flow voids on T2 WI

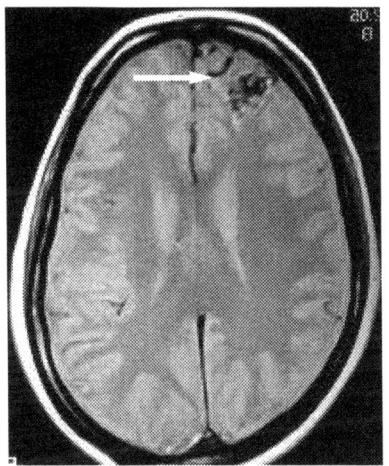 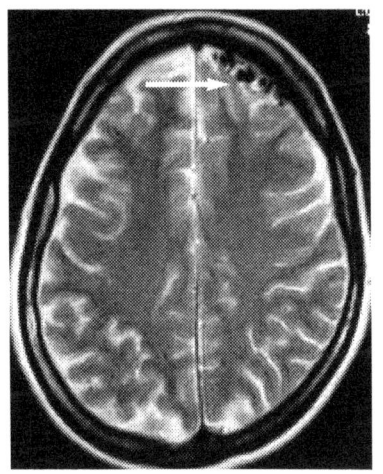

Figure 48. *The image on the left is an uncontrasted axial T1 WI and the image on the right an axial T2 WI. They both demonstrate the serpentine flow voids (arrows) associated with an arteriovenous malformation.*

Cavernous Malformation (multiple in > 50%, also called cavernoma)
CT scan
Small hyperdense mass
Little or no enhancement
MR scan
'Popcorn' lesion - multi lobulated
Variable intensity depending on age of haematoma with hypointense, siderotic rim on T2 WI
Little or no enhancement

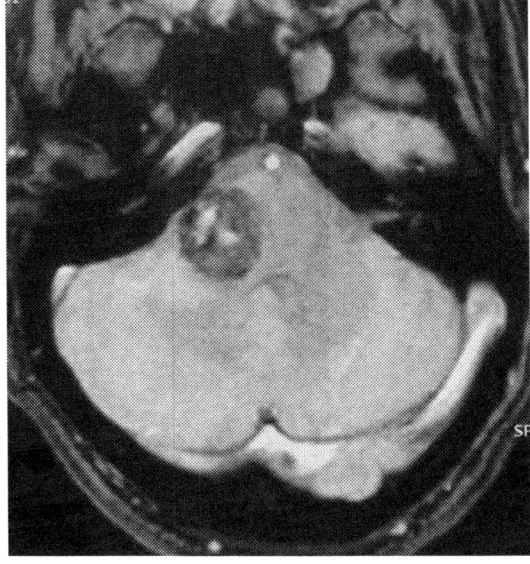

Figure 49. *This is an axial T2 WI. This brainstem cavernoma demonstrates the typical 'popcorn' appearance and has a siderotic, black ring around it.*

Venous angioma
CT scan
Usually normal
Small enhancing mass
MR scan
Variable intensity depending flow and on age of associated haematoma
Caput medusae lesion with several veins draining to single large vein
Central hypodense centre on T1 WI

Infection

Empyema
CT scan (can miss lesion)
Can be subdural or extradural
Enhancing rim
Frequently spreads from infection in mastoids and facial sinuses
MR scan (much more sensitive, especially coronal cuts)
More intense signal than CSF on T1 WI
Enhances strongly
Underlying brain hyperintense on T2 WI due to reactive, oedematous brain

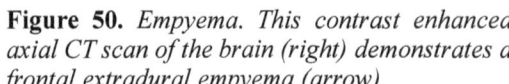

Figure 50. *Empyema. This contrast enhanced axial CT scan of the brain (right) demonstrates a frontal extradural empyema (arrow).*

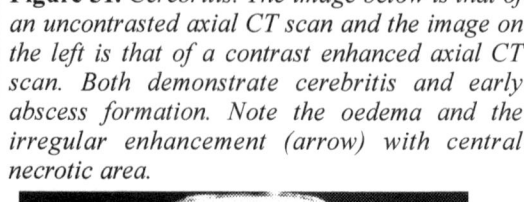

Figure 51. *Cerebritis. The image below is that of an uncontrasted axial CT scan and the image on the left is that of a contrast enhanced axial CT scan. Both demonstrate cerebritis and early abscess formation. Note the oedema and the irregular enhancement (arrow) with central necrotic area.*

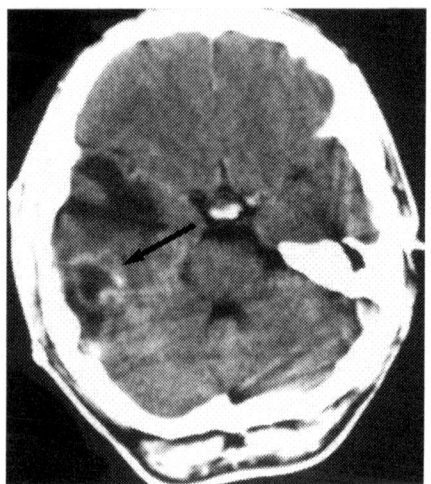

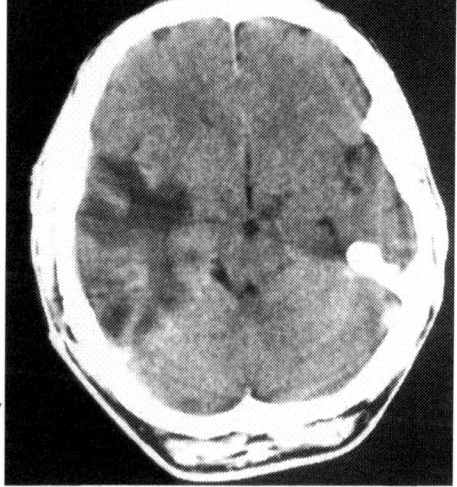

Cerebritis
CT scan
Hypodensity, surrounding oedema
Enhances strongly but inhomogeneously with contrast
MR scan
Hypodense, inhomogeneous on T1 WI
Hyperintense T2 WI
Enhances with contrast

Abscess
CT scan
Central hypodensity
Capsule, thinnest on the aspect facing the ventricle
Capsule enhances strongly and uniformly
Surrounding oedema
MR scan

Hyperintense T2 WI
Capsule enhances strongly and uniformly
Surrounding oedema

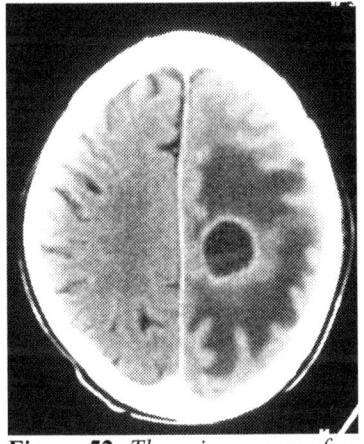
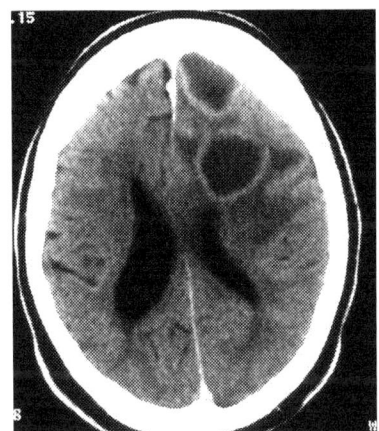

Figure 52. *These images are from axial contrast enhanced CT scans and the image on the left demonstrates a single abscess with associated oedema. The image on the right demonstrates two abscesses.*

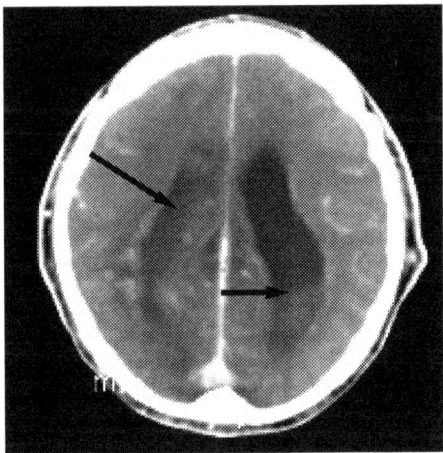

Figure 53. *This contrast enhanced axial CT scan of the brain demonstrates severe intracranial infection. The image demonstrates ventriculitis with pus in the right lateral ventricle leading to a cast in the ventricle (top arrow) as well as pus in the left lateral ventricle as demonstrated by the fluid-fluid level (bottom arrow).*

4

SPINAL IMAGING

Contents

Normal appearances of spinal MR imaging

Clearing C-spine X-rays following trauma

Degenerative conditions
Rheumatoid arthritis
Spinal stenosis
Disc herniation

Spinal tumours

Extradural compartment
Primary tumours
Bony tumours and cartilage producing tumours of the spine
Osteoid osteoma
Osteoblastoma
Osteochondroma
Lymphoproliferative tumours
Solitary plasmacytoma
Multiple myeloma
Lymphoma
Tumour of notochordal origin
Chordoma
Metastatic tumours

Intradural, extramedullary compartment
Meningioma
Schwannoma
Myxopapillary ependymoma

Intramedullary compartment
Ependymoma
Astrocytoma
Paraganglioma
Haemangioblastoma
Cysts
Arachnoid cyst
Dermoid cyst
Epidermoid cyst
Perineural cyst (Tarlov cyst)

Synovial cyst
Neurenteric cyst

Infection
Osteomyelitis
Epidural empyema (abscess)
Discitis
Tuberculosis of the spine

Vascular pathology
Abnormal vasculature
Dural arteriovenous fistula
Arteriovenous malformation
Cavernous angioma
Spinal cord infarct
Subdural haematoma
Epidural haematoma

Normal appearances of the spine on MR imaging
Vertebrae
Vertebral bodies are hyperintense compared to spinal cord on T1 WI with the marrow (containing fat) being more intense than the rest of the vertebra. The vertebrae are of a slightly higher intensity that the intervertebral discs on T1 WI. The hallmark of pathology in vertebrae is a decrease on T1 WI and an increase of intensity on T2 WI due to the increased water content associated with most pathology and the displacement of the normal marrow.

Neural foramina
When evaluating sagittal MR scans as in figure 1, the scout view will orientate you as to whether the image is to the right or the left of the midline. The upper portion of the neural foramen contains fatty connective tissue with the nerve root located in the inferior portion of the foramen. The nerve root will be displaced in lateral disc protrusions and may be displaced upwards, displacing the fatty tissue.

Intervertebral disc
Healthy discs in young patients have a high water content and therefore are hypointense on T1 WI and relatively hyperintense on T2 WI. As patients get older, the discs dehydrate or they may dehydrate secondary to pathological processes, becoming relatively hypointense on T2 WI compared to normal discs. The annulus fibrous appears as a hypointense signal on T1WI and T2 WI.

Spinal cord
All neural tissues demonstrate intermediate signal intensity (gray) on both T1 and T2 WI. CSF demonstrates hypointensity on T1 WI and is hyperintense on T2 WI.

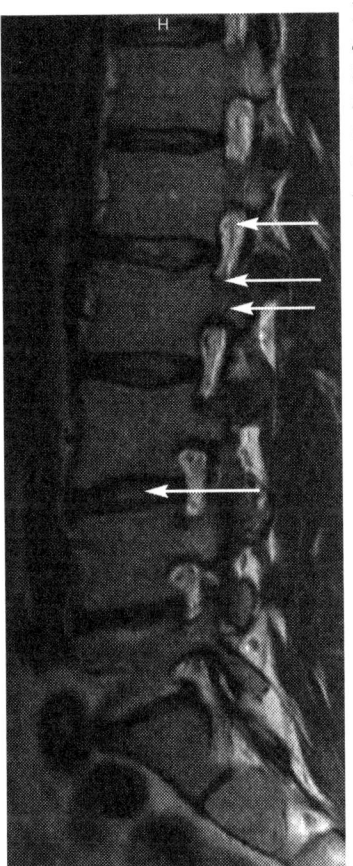

Figure 1. *This is a sagittal T2 WI of the lumbosacral spine. This image is taken off the midline, and in this case to the right of the spinal canal, and demonstrates the neural foramina, which are white due to the fatty tissue contained within them. The top arrow points toward the top of a neural foramen and the next arrow to the bottom. Note that this arrow points directly at the nerve as it lies in the inferior part of the foramen. The third arrow points directly at a pedicle. The last arrow points at an intervertebral disc.*

Clearing C-spine X-rays following trauma
The following three views are essential and mandatory:
Lateral c-spine film demonstrating the C7-T1 junction clearly and demonstrating the upper border of T1. If this is not possible with a normal lateral film, then a swimmers view should be performed (one arm above the head).
A-P view
Open mouth view demonstrating the odontoid process.

The following sequence is useful in clearing the cervical spine:
Alignment – Assess the alignment of the anterior vertebral line, the posterior vertebral line and the spinolaminar line. More than 3.5 mm subluxation is abnormal. At C2/C3 there may be a normal physiological subluxation of up to 3mm, especially in children. Subluxation of up to 50% of the width of the vertebral body signifies unifacet dislocation and a subluxation of more than this signifies a bifacet dislocation, which is usually accompanied by widening of the interspinous spaces.
Angulation – angulation of more than 11 degrees between two adjacent vertebrae is indicative of a fracture or ligamentous injury and potential instability.
The diameter of the spinal canal – anything less than 14 mm is indicative of impending spinal cord compression.
Examination of the pre vertebral soft tissue shadow - from C1 to C4 the soft tissue should be maximally half the width of a vertebral body and below C4 it should be maximally equal to the width of a vertebral body (5mm at C2 and 17 - 22 mm at C6).

The distance between the skull base and the atlas should not exceed 5mm as this can be indicative of atlanto – occipital dissociation.

The vertebral bodies should be examined to ascertain that there are no compression fractures or burst fractures.

The intervertebral discs are not visible on plain x-rays or CT scans but they can be examined by looking at the disc spaces between the vertebrae which demonstrate the anatomy of the (invisible) discs. Therefore a narrowing of one disc space will imply that there has been compression, and possibly herniation, of an intervertebral disc. If there is an associated neurological deficit without a fracture or dislocation, an MR scan will demonstrate the anatomy of the disc and any related prolapse.

The odontoid peg should be examined on the open mouth view for fractures. The vertical line that separates the front teeth must not be confused with a fracture. On the lateral c-spine view there should not be more than 3mm between the dens and the atlas (atlanto-dens interval). More than this implies injury to the transverse ligament and more than 5mm implies disruption of this ligament.

Degenerative conditions
Rheumatoid arthritis
CT scanning may demonstrate C1/2 subluxation, cranial settling and dens erosions. MRI may demonstrate pannus formation and acquired spinal stenosis. Plain flexion and extension images as well as MR in flexion and extension are invaluable to demonstrate dynamic subluxations.

Spinal stenosis
Spinal stenosis is either congenital or acquired. Sagittal T2 WI demonstrates spinal stenosis well but the most useful image is the axial T2 WI. In the cervical spine, anterior compression of the spinal cord can be caused by prolapsed discs, osteophytic bars, ossification of the posterior longitudinal ligament, subluxation of the vertebrae and vertebral compression fractures. Posterior and lateral compression can be caused by hypertrophy of the ligamentum flavum and the facet joints. Damage to the cord is shown as hyperintensity on the T2 WI. In the lumbar spine the classic trefoil shape can be seen with the round canal taking on a triangular shape. There is usually encroachment due to facet joint hypertrophy as well as thickened ligamentum flavum. Added stenosis is caused by degrees of vertebral body subluxation and plain film extension and flexion views are important in identifying whether this is stable or not.

Disc herniation (prolapse)
The best images to evaluate the presence of disc herniation are the T2 WI as the CSF, being brilliantly white, contrasts well with the rest of the tissue and demonstrating a disc protrusion is easier than on T1WI where the intensity of the tissues are frequently quite similar. The best approach is to look at the sagittal T2 WI and pinpoint the pathology. Then use the axial T2 WI to evaluate the extent of the neural compromise. The T1 WI are good for evaluating the intervertebral foramina and looking at fine detail of the nervous structures. The sagittal and coronal images are useful for evaluating the lateral elements.

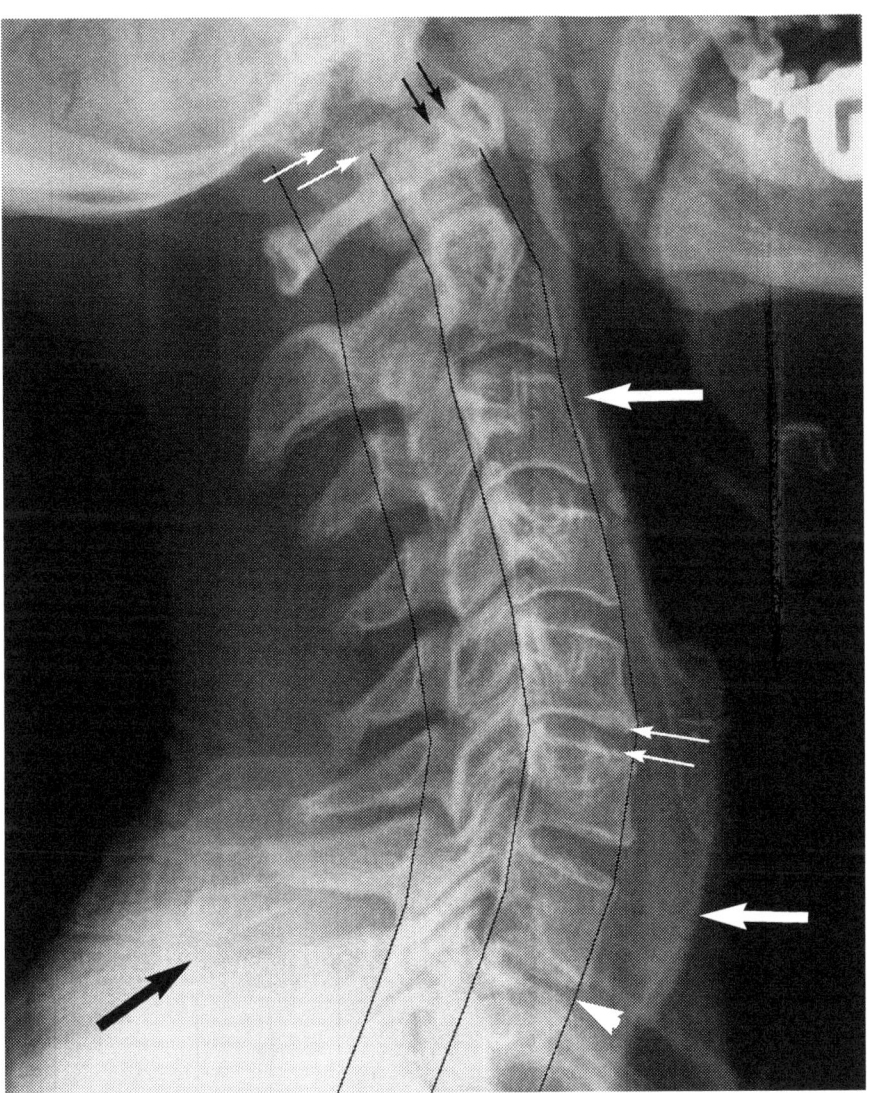

Figure 2. *This image depicts a lateral cervical spine x-ray. The two thin black arrows at the skull base demonstrates the atlanto-dens interval which should not exceed 3mm. The two thin white arrows demonstrate the space between the top of the atlas and the base of the skull which should not exceed 5mm. The top thick white arrow demonstrates the pre vertebral soft tissue shadow from C1 to C4 and the bottom thick white arrow the soft tissue below C4. The soft tissue from C1 to C4 should be maximally half the width of a vertebral body and below C4 it should be maximally equal to the width of a vertebral body (5mm at C2 and 17 - 22 mm at C6). The bottom two thin white arrows point toward a narrowed C5/6 disc space. MRI confirmed a C5/6 disc prolapse. The thick white arrow head points at the top edge of T1 which must always be seen. The thick black arrow points toward a clay shoveler's fracture (avulsion fracture of the tip of the spinous process). Note the three lines (anterior vertebral line, the posterior vertebral line and the spinolaminar line) demonstrating the alignment of the cervical spine.*

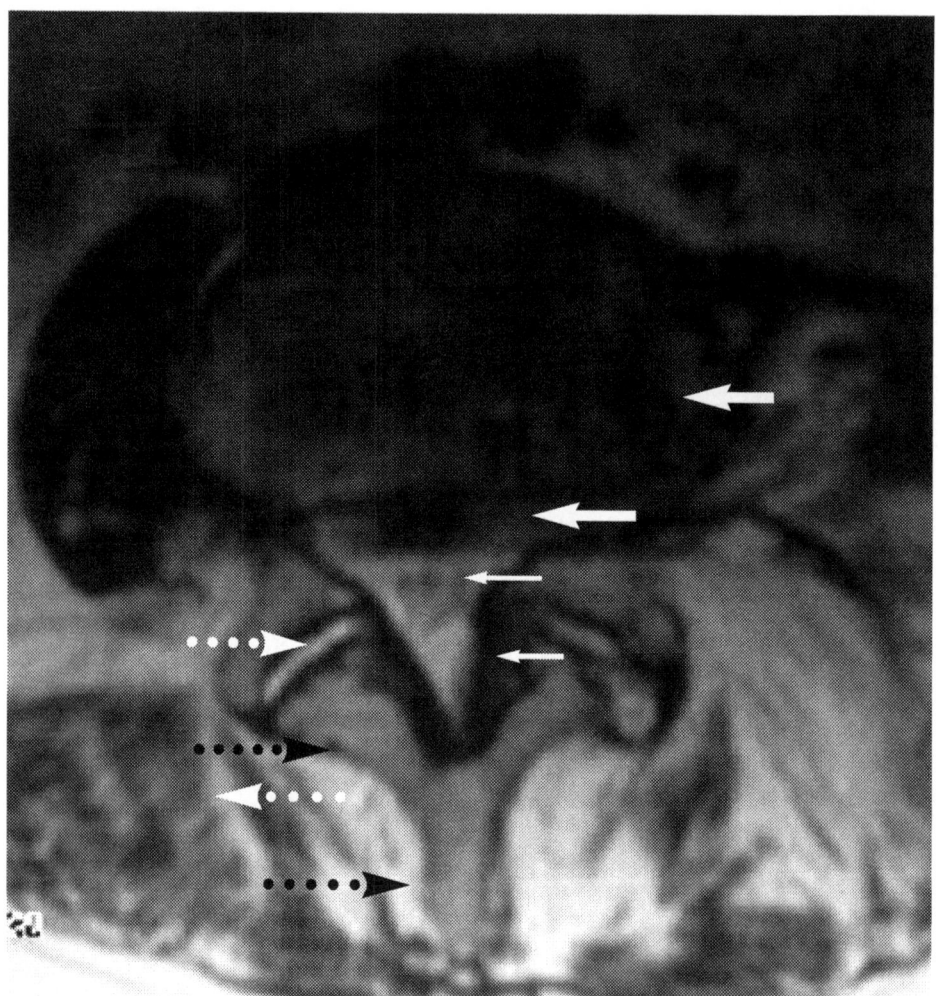

Figure 3. *This is an axial T2 WI of the lumbar spine demonstrating spinal stenosis. The top thick white arrow demonstrates the intervertebral disc. The next thick white arrow demonstrates a broad, flat central disc prolapse. The top thin white arrow demonstrates the compressed cauda equina, which takes on a trefoil shape. The bottom thin white arrow demonstrates the thickened and hypertrophied ligamentum flavum that is a main contributing factor in spinal stenosis. The top dashed white arrow demonstrates the facet joint, the bottom dashed white arrow demonstrates the paraspinal muscles, the top dashed black arrow demonstrates the lamina on the right-hand side and bottom dashed black arrow demonstrates the spinous process.*

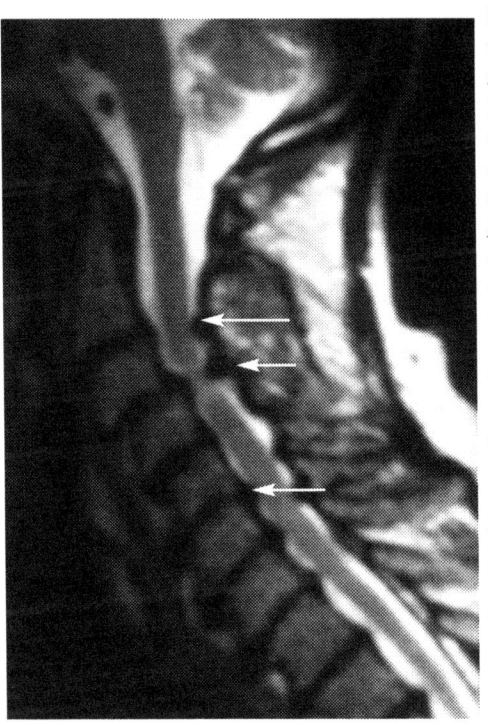

Figure 4. This is a sagittal T2 WI of the cervical spine in a patient with severe cervical spondylosis and clinical quadri spasticity. The top arrow is pointing at a thickened area of ligamentum flavum, as is the next arrow down. The third arrow points toward anterior compression from a disc-osteophyte complex. Note how this patient has both severe anterior and posterior compression of the spinal cord. The intervertebral discs have associated bony osteophytes which are hard and require extensive drilling at the time of surgery. The decision as to whether a decompression is done from an anterior or posterior approach is based on where the compression is and how many levels are affected. Up to three levels may be decompressed from anterior with anterior cervical discectomies or corpectomies. A posterior approach via laminectomy is usually performed for extensive disease. Flexion and extension X-rays are useful to decide whether fusion is required at the same time.

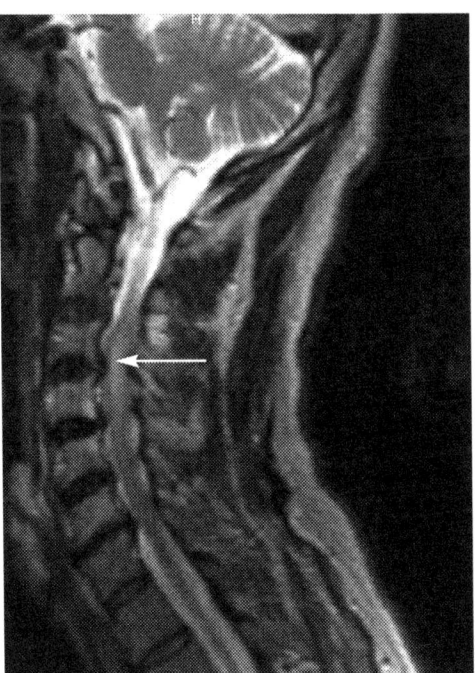

Figure 5. This sagittal T2 WI of the cervical spine in a different patient from above, also demonstrates severe cervical spondylosis. The arrow is pointing towards associated signal change in the cord, which is a poor prognostic sign.

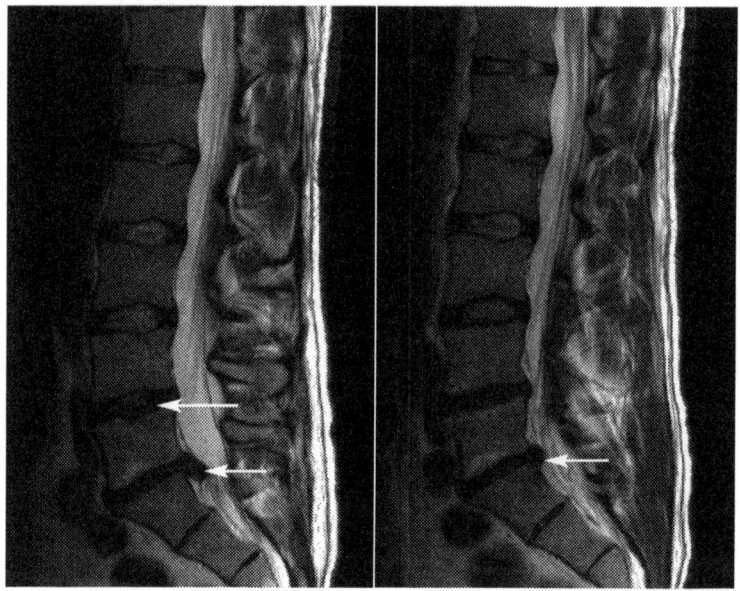

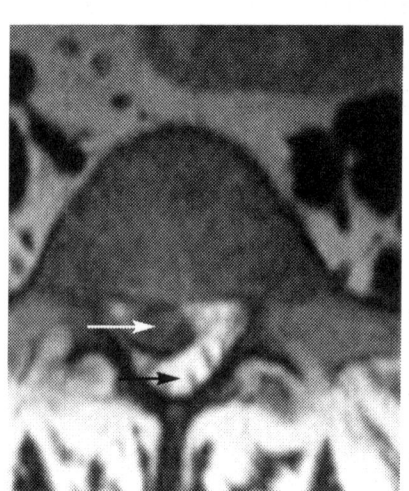

Figure 6. *The top images are sagittal T2 WI and the image on the left is an axial T2 WI of the same patient. The top arrow on the top left image demonstrates a degenerative intervertebral disc. Note how the intensity has changed from the normal intervertebral discs above it. This lower intensity is due to a lower water content of this damaged disc. The next arrow down shows a large downward extrusion of an intervertebral disc. The image top right is an image slightly towards the right of the midline compared to the image on the left. Note how the herniated segment appears smaller. This is because this is a mostly central disc prolapse as is demonstrated in the image on the left by the white arrow. The black arrow demonstrates the cauda equina which is compressed by the disc fragment*

Spinal tumours

Extradural compartment

PRIMARY TUMOURS

Bony tumours and cartilage producing tumours of the spine
Osteoid osteoma
CT scan
Hypodense nucleus, with surrounding sclerosis, may have associated calcium
Lesion is less than 1.5 cm in diameter
May enhance with contrast
MR scan
Hypointense on T1 WI and hyperintense on T2 WI
Calcium leads to hypointensity on both T1 and T2 WI sequences.

Osteoblastoma
CT scan
Hypodense nucleus, may have associated calcium, surrounding sclerosis as in osteoid osteoma
Lesion is more than 1.5 cm in diameter
It is an obviously expansile lesion
May enhance with contrast
Evidence of infiltration and destruction
MR scan
Hypointense on T1 WI and hyperintense on T2 WI
Surrounding oedema and may have soft tissue component

Osteochondroma
CT scan
A sessile bony outcrop with a cartilage cap
The cap may contain calcium
MR scan
On T1 WI a hyperintense centre (marrow) surrounded by a hypointense rim (cortex) and hypointense/isointense cap (cartilage).
On T2 WI an isointense centre (marrow) surrounded by a hypointense rim (cortex) and a hyperintense cap (cartilage)

Lymphoproliferative tumours
Solitary plasmacytoma
CT scan
Solitary lytic destructive lesion with collapse of the vertebra
May have soft tissue mass
Does not enhance
MR scan
Solitary lesion, hypo/isointense on T1 WI
Involves posterior elements with vertebral collapse
Moderate enhancement after gadolinium on T1 WI
Heterogeneous signal on T2 WI

Multiple myeloma
MR scan
This is a multifocal disease of the marrow of vertebrae with patchy involvement demonstrated on T1 WI as hypointense areas and on T2 WI as hyperintense areas.
Moderate enhancement after gadolinium on T1 WI

Lymphoma
CT scan
Homogeneous epidural mass
Enhances homogeneously with contrast
May present as lytic osseous lesion with associated soft tissue mass
MR scan
Homogenous epidural mass isointense on T1 WI with intense, homogeneous enhancement after contrast administration and hyperintense on T2 WI
May appear with characteristics as above but in the intramedullary space
May present as osseous lesion, hypointense on T1 WI with contrast enhancement and hyperintense on T2 WI

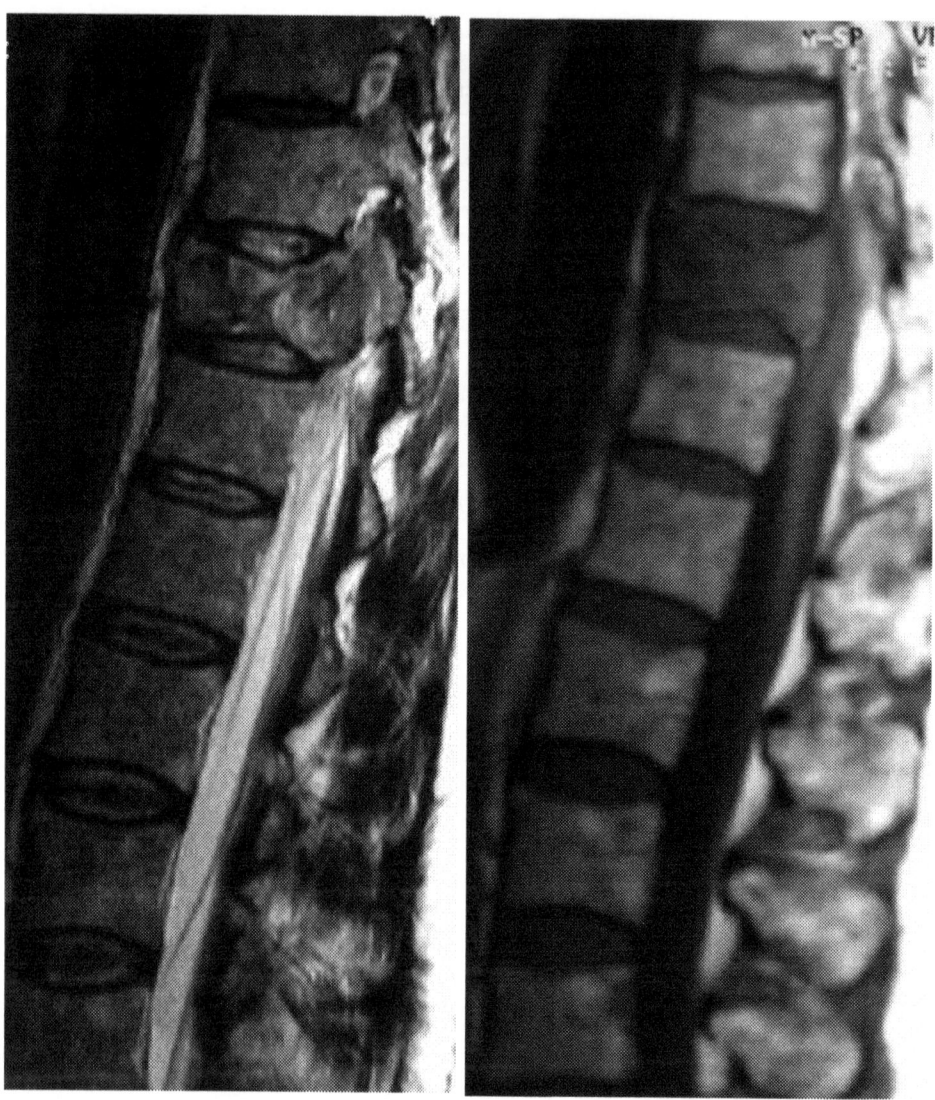

Figure 7. *The image on the left is a sagittal T2 WI of the thoracic spine and the image on the right is a sagittal T1 WI of the thoracic spine, both demonstrating a multiple myeloma lesion. Note how this lesion is centered on the anterior aspect of the vertebral body and extends into the spinal canal. The lesion is isointense to slightly hyperintense on T2 WI and hypointense on T1 WI*

Tumours of notochordal origin
Chordoma
CT scan
Destructive lytic lesion with associated soft tissue mass
Contains calcium and sclerotic elements
Enhances heterogeneously with contrast
MR scan
Heterogenous mass, hypointense on T1 WI with heterogeneous enhancement after contrast and hyperintense on T2 WI

METASTATIC TUMOURS (prostate, breast adenocarcinoma, lung adenocarcinoma, renal cell carcinoma and gastric carcinoma)
CT scan
Lytic, permeative lesion found mostly in posterior vertebral body but also pedicle and rest of vertebral body
May have associated soft tissue mass and may enhance with contrast.
MR scan
Disc sparing involvement of the vertebrae with vertebral destruction and may be associated with vertebral body collapse
On T1 WI the tumours are hypointense to bone and enhancement is variable
On T2 WI the tumours are hypo/isointense to marrow.

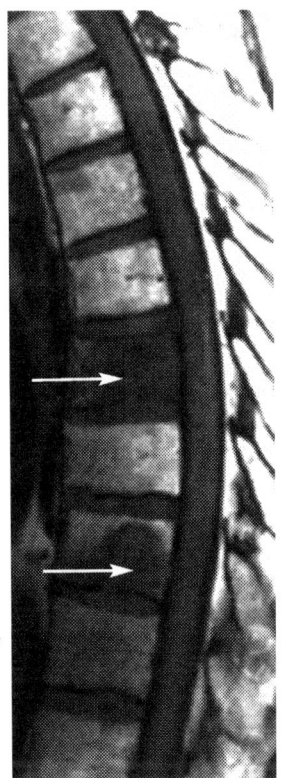

Figure 8. *This is a sagittal T1 WI of the thoracic spine which demonstrates two thoracic metastatic lesions. These vertebrae are darker in colour because the disease process has led to an increased water content of the affected vertebrae. Both vertebrae are still intact and have not lost their integrity. It is common for the vertebrae to collapse. Note the sparing of the relatively avascular intervertebral discs.*

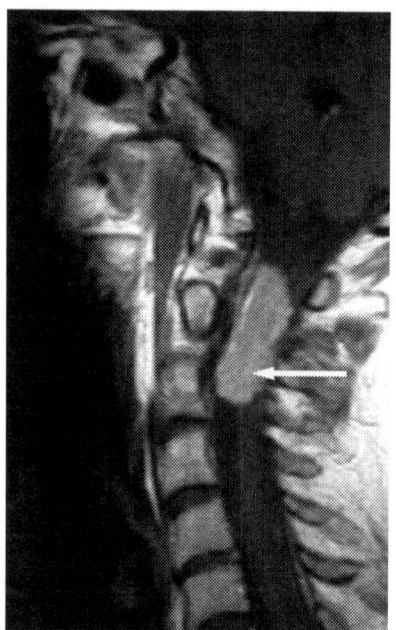
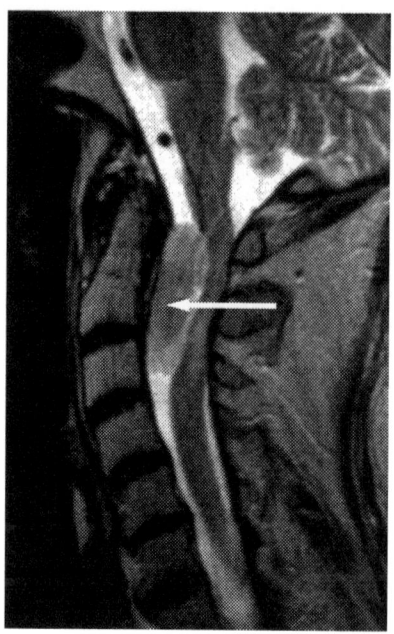
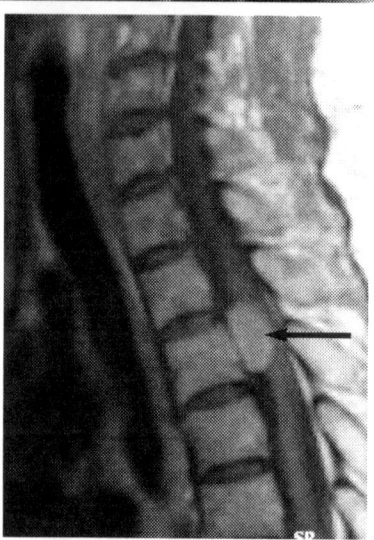

Figure 9. *The image on the top left is a sagittal contrast enhanced T1 WI of the cervical spine and the image top right is a sagittal T2 WI of the cervical spine. Both demonstrate a meningioma. Note how the meningioma is hyperintense to spinal cord following contrast enhancement and hyperintense to cord on the T2 WI. On T1 WI pre contrast these lesions are usually iso/hypointense to the tissue of the spinal cord. The image on the left is a sagittal T1 WI with contrast enhancement demonstrating a meningioma in the thoracic spinal canal.*

Intradural, extramedullary compartment

Meningioma
CT scan
Iso/hyperdense mass that enhances homogeneously with contrast
MR scan
Isointense to cord on T1 WI with intense homogeneous enhancement following contrast administration
Iso/hyperintense on T2 WI

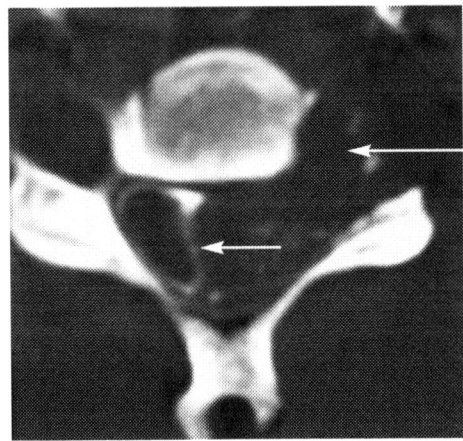

Figure 10. *This axial CT scan of the cervical spine demonstrates a neurofibroma that is extending through an expanded neural foramen on the left (top arrow). The spinal cord is completely pushed over to the other side (bottom arrow) and the neurofibroma fills nearly the whole of the spinal canal.*

Schwannoma
MR scan
Isointense to cord on T1 WI with intense homogeneous enhancement
Hyperintense on T2 WI
May have dumbbell extension through neural foramina

Myxopapillary ependymoma (arises in the conus medullaris or filum terminale)
CT scan
There may be evidence of spinal canal widening or pedicle erosion in the area of the conus
MR scan
This is frequently a heterogeneous lesion. They are usually isointense to cord on T1 WI with intense and well-delineated homogeneous enhancement and hyperintense on T2 WI There is an 80% incidence of associated cysts either within the tumour, rostral or caudal cysts at the poles of the tumour or reactive dilatation of the central canal.

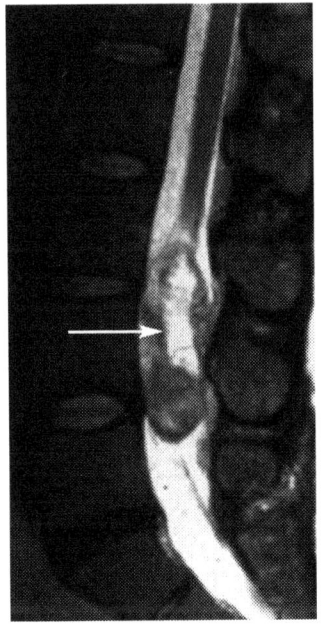

Figure 11. *This sagittal T2 WI of the lumbosacral spine demonstrates a myxopapillary ependymoma of the conus medullaris. Note the heterogeneous appearance and the hyperintense cyst fluid (arrow). This lesion expands the cord circumferentialy outwards.*

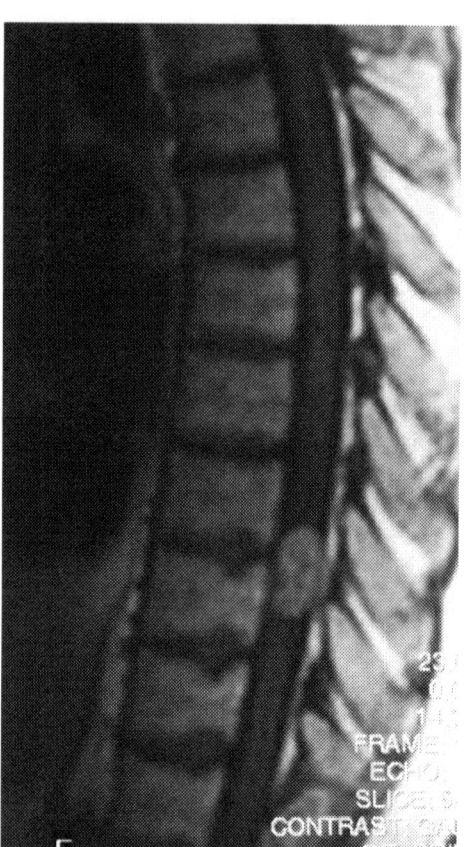

Figure 12. *This is a contrast enhanced T1 WI demonstrating a neurofibroma of the thoracic spine. Note how these lesions are very similar in appearance to the intraspinal meningiomas.*

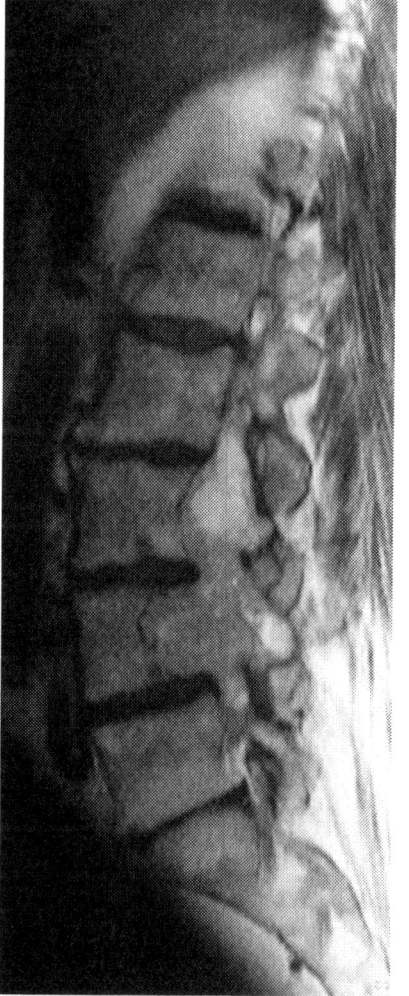

Figure 13. *This sagittal T2 WI of the lumbosacral spine demonstrates a heterogeneous hyperintense lesion. This paraganglioma proved to be extremely vascular at surgery*

Intramedullary compartment

Ependymoma (55% of intramedullary tumours)
CT scan
There may be evidence of spinal canal widening or pedicle erosion
MR scan
Isointense to cord on T1 WI with intense and well-delineated homogeneous enhancement (much better than the patchy enhancement seen with astrocytomas of the cord). Hyperintense on T2 WI, may be heterogeneous. Since they arise from the ependyma that lines the central canal, they are usually centrally located.

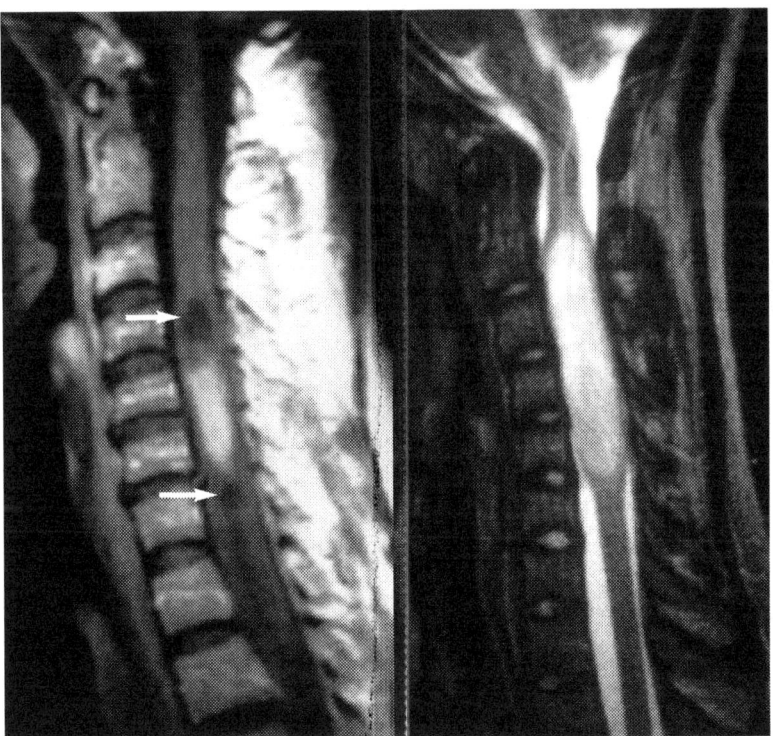

Figure 14. *The image on the left is a sagittal contrast enhanced T1 WI of the cervical spine that demonstrates an ependymoma. Note the two polar cysts as demonstrated by the two arrows. The lesion enhances homogeneously and intensely with contrast. The image on the right is a sagittal T2 WI of the cervical spine and demonstrates an ependymoma. It is homogeneous and hyperintense with good demarcation and is seen to expand the cord.*

Astrocytoma (30% of intramedullary tumours)
CT scan
There may be evidence of spinal canal widening or pedicle erosion
MR scan
Expanded cord that may have cystic component on T1 WI with variable signal intensity and variable enhancement and is hyperintense on T2 WI. These lesions appear very similar to the ependymomas. They arise from the parenchyma of the cord and are more eccentrically located than ependymomas.

Paraganglioma
CT scan
There may be evidence of spinal canal widening or pedicle erosion
MR scan
Well delineated mass hypo/isointense on T1 WI with intense homogeneous enhancement
Hyperintense on T2 WI

Haemangioblastoma
CT scan
There may be evidence of spinal canal widening or pedicle erosion
MR scan
Well delineated cystic mass hypo/isointense on T1 WI with enhancing nodule.
Hyperintense on T2 WI. May have associated syringomyelia.

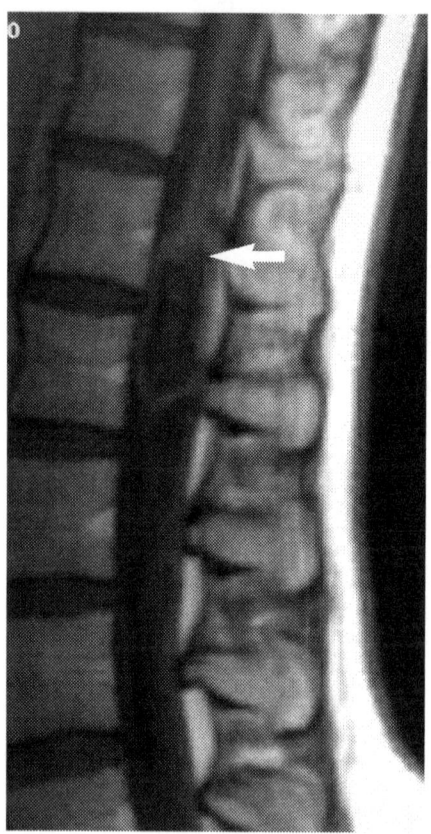 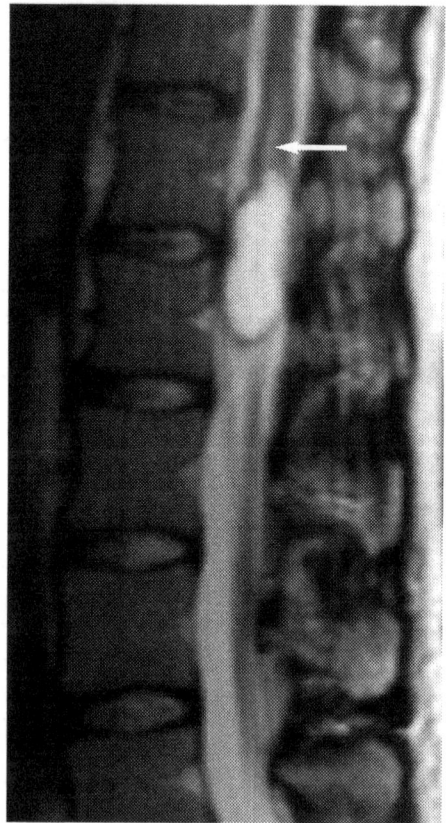

Figure 15. *Haemangioblastoma. The image on the left is a sagittal uncontrasted T1 WI of the thoracic spine and the image on the right is a sagittal T2 WI of the thoracic spine. Note the cystic mass with the mural nodule (thick arrow). This nodule enhanced with the administration of contrast. Note the associated syringomyelia (thin arrow).*

Cysts

Arachnoid cyst
MR scan
Extramedullary mass in either intra – or extradural space, CSF density (hypointense on T1 WI and hyperintense on T2 WI)
No contrast enhancement
Supresses on FLAIR images

Dermoid cyst (located in midline)
MR scan
Hyperintense on T1 WI (hypointense on STIR)
Heterogenous on T2 WI
May enhance

Epidermoid cyst (located in midline)
MR scan
Hypointense on T1 WI
Hyperintense on T2 WI
Does not suppress on FLAIR sequence

Perineural cyst (Tarlov cyst)
MR scan
A cystic enlargement of the nerve root sleeve, collection of CSF between the endoneurium and perineurium of the nerve root
Well defined with CSF intensity – hypointense on T1 WI and hyperintense on T2 WI

Synovial cyst
MR scan
Outpouching from the facet joint
Well defined with variable intensity secondary to protein contents
Enhancing rim

Neurenteric cyst
MR scan
Intradural, extramedullary cyst or intramedullary cysts
Isointense or slightly hyperintense to cerebrospinal fluid on T1 WI and hyperintense on T2 WI (fluid containing a high protein content within the cyst)
Associated vertebral abnormalities
Focal atrophy of the cord secondary from chronic compressive effect

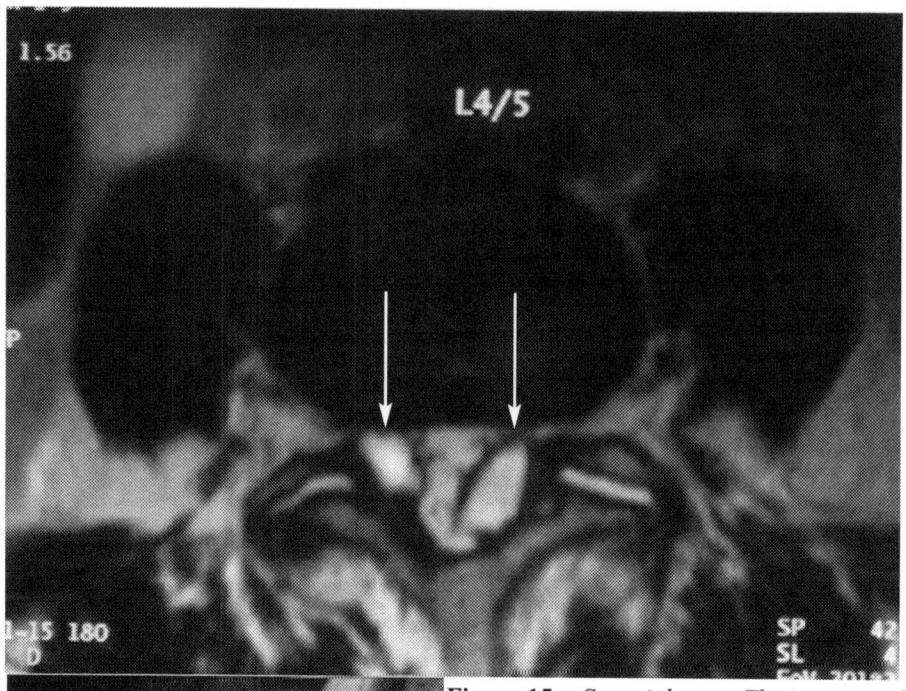

Figure 15a. Synovial cysts. The image on the top is an axial T2 WI and the image on the left is a sagittal T2 WI. Note how the cysts are hyperintense and appear to arise from the facet joint.

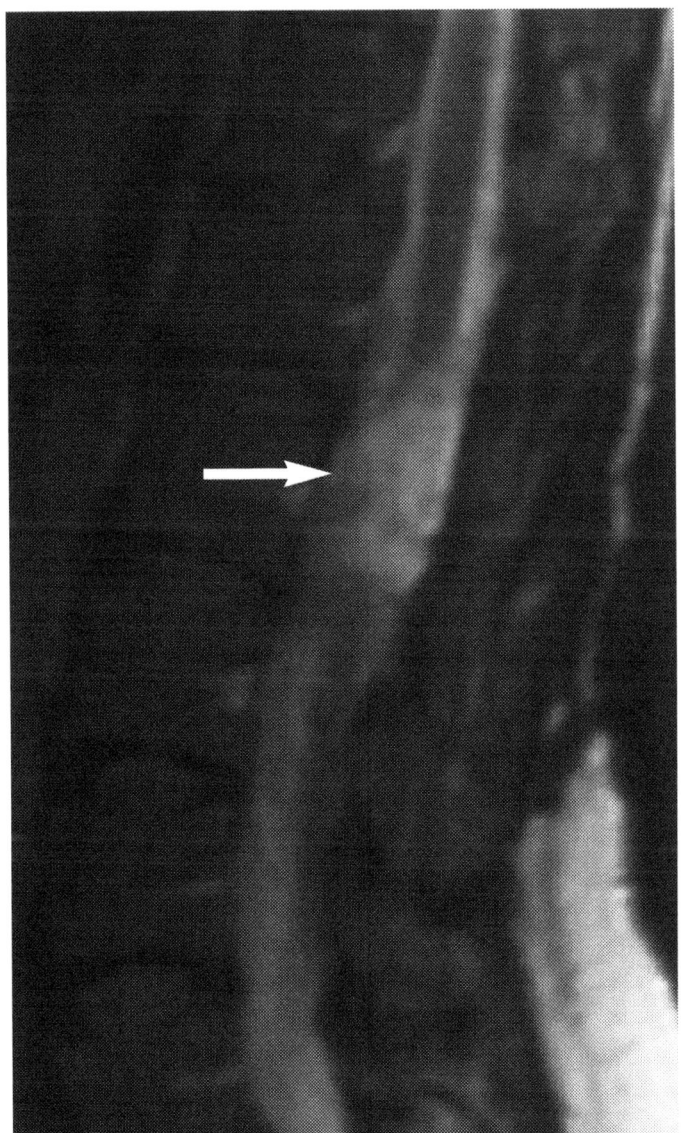

Figure 15b. *Dermoid cyst. The image is a sagittal T2 WI. Note how the cyst is hyperintense and heterogeneous. It would also be hyperintense on T1 WI. Fat suppression sequences like a STIR sequence will suppress the signal of the tumour.*

Infection
Osteomyelitis
Computer tomography is sensitive for detecting infection in the vertebrae, showing hypodensity at the site as well as frequently showing gas within the vertebrae. Associated discitis will lead to hypodensity of the infected discs. When there is healing of the lesions in the chronic phase the lesions become denser. On MRI scan there are low intensity changes on T1 WI and high intensity changes on T2 WI because of the increased water content and the lesions frequently enhance with contrast.

Epidural empyema (abscess)

MRI scanning of the spine is the imaging of choice showing a hypointense lesion on T1 WI that is hyperintense on T2 WI and enhances with contrast. The anterior located collections are almost always associated with discitis. Radionuclide scans are extremely sensitive and are usually the first imaging modality to detect these lesions.

Discitis

On imaging the disc appears hypointense on T1 WI and hyperintense on T2 WI, demonstrating a higher fluid content and may enhance with Gadolinium contrast administration.

Tuberculosis of the spine

Infection with *mycobacterium tuberculosis* starts in the vertebra or adjacent endplate and its hallmark is destruction of the vertebra and gibbus formation with collapse of the vertebra, whilst the integrity of the disc is maintained until quite late in the disease. On x-ray vertebral involvement with erosion kyphosis, with mostly involvement of the vertebrae and sparing the posterior elements is seen. There is frequently some soft tissue involvement with calcification. CT scans are quite useful in delineating the extent of the disease and demonstrating bony involvement and bony sequestra. MR may demonstrate as associated cold psoas abscess. Typically, the intervertebral disc is spared with the gibbus hypointense on T1 WI and hyperintense on T2 WI.

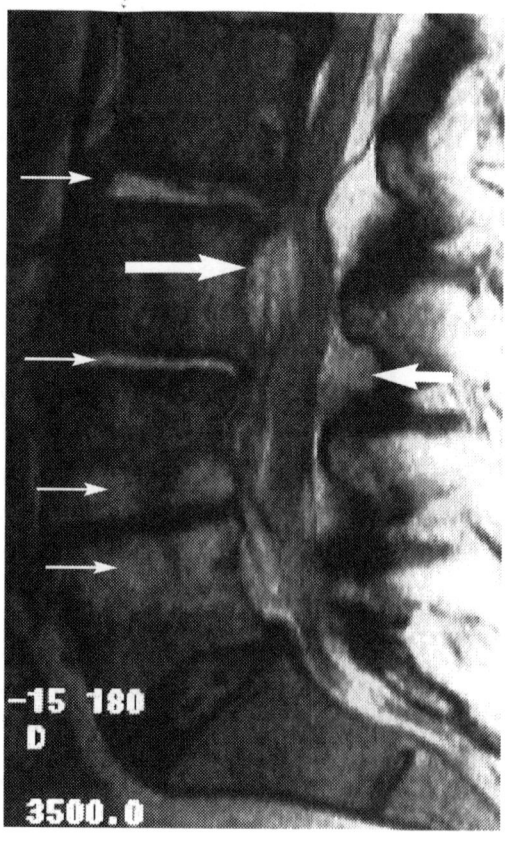

Figure 16. *This is a sagittal T2 WI of the lumbosacral spine. The two thick arrows demonstrate collections of pus, one anterior and one posterior of the cauda equina. The two top thin arrows demonstrate discitis with increased signal intensity. This is due to oedema associated with the infection of these disc spaces. The two bottom arrows demonstrate increased signal intensity in the vertebrae adjacent to the disc space signalling osteomyelitis.*

Vascular pathology
Abnormal vasculature
Dural Arteriovenous fistula (Type I AVM)
Usually located in the posterior intradural space either in or adjacent to the intervertebral foramen and is fed by a single arterial feeder entering the dural space through a dural root sleeve. On T1 WI the cord may be enlarged with multiple enhancing pial vessels and on T2 WI the cord is also enlarged with flow voids in the pia on the surface of the cord.

Arteriovenous malformation - Type II, III and IV (Type 1 is a dural AVF)
Type II has a nidus in the intramedullary space. Type III has an intramedullary nidus but with extramedullary extension and type IV is located ventrally, intra durally and perimedullary. Type II and III (intramedullary) demonstrate an enlarged cord and heterogenous signal on T1 WI and contrast enhancement. On T2 WI these are hyperintense and contain flow voids. Type IV demonstrates a ventral fistula with prominent flow voids on T1 WI and T2 WI demonstrates a hyperintense ventral lesion with flow voids.

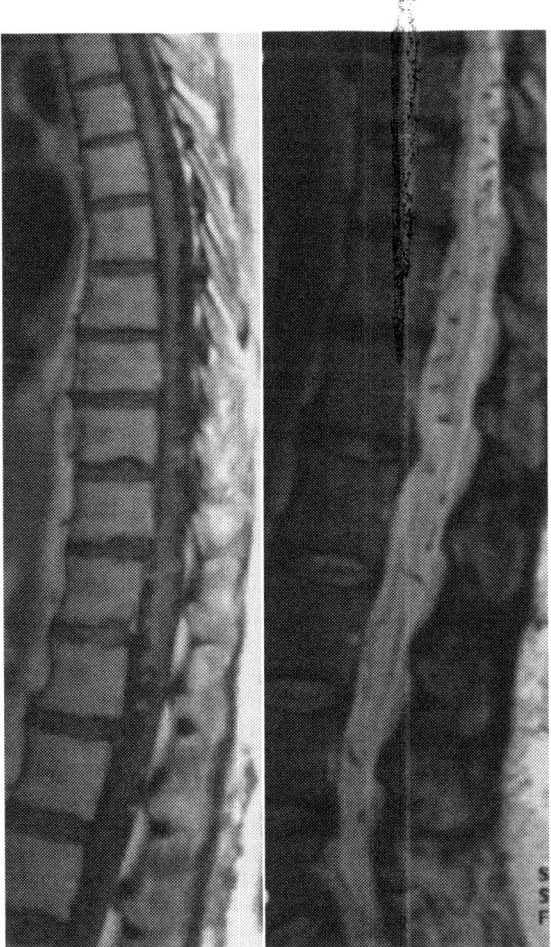

Figure 17. *The image on the left is a sagittal T1 WI and the image on the right is a sagittal T2 WI of the spine. Both demonstrate extensive flow voids from a arteriovenous malformation. The true nature of the vascular supply and drainage would be obtained from spinal angiography.*

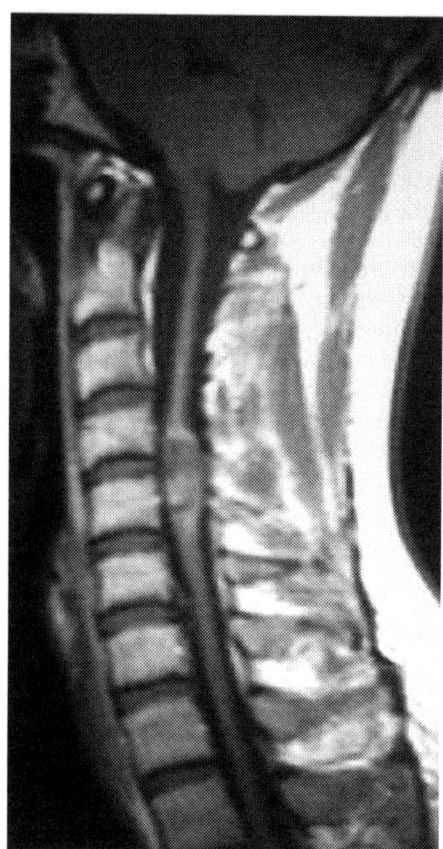 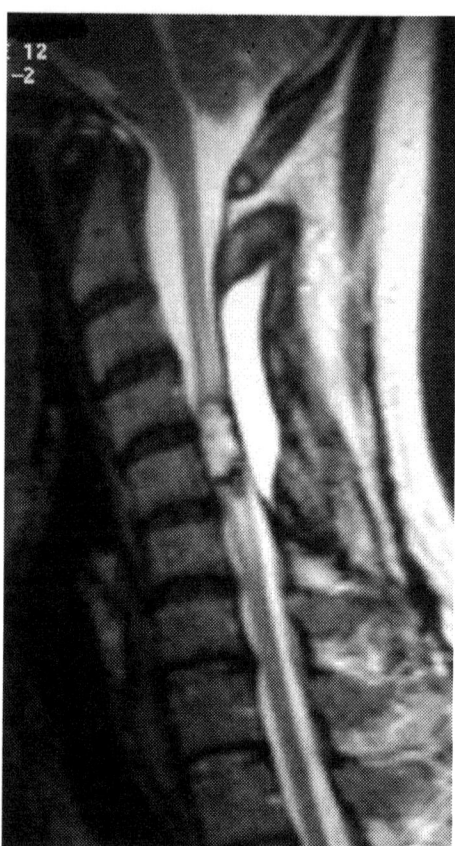

Figure 18. *Cavernoma. The image on the left is a sagittal contrast enhanced T1 WI of the cervical spine and the image on the right is a sagittal T2 WI of the cervical spine. Note the lobulated appearance of the lesion and the black, siderotic rim on the T2 WI.*

Cavernous angioma (cavernous malformation, cavernoma)
These intramedullary lesions have heterogenous signal on T1 and T2 WI with a hypodense ring (hemosiderin) on T2 WI.

Spinal cord infarct
The cord is usually slightly swollen but may be normal diameter and on T1 WI it usually has no features and on T2 WI is hyperintense to spinal cord. There may be a focal haemorrhagic conversion of the infarct.

Subdural haematoma
On CT scans these lesions are hyperdense in the acute and subacute phases. On MR scanning the intensity varies (see chapter 5) and it can be difficult to distinguish the blood from normal CSF. There might be some displacement of the cord that may be helpful in diagnosis.

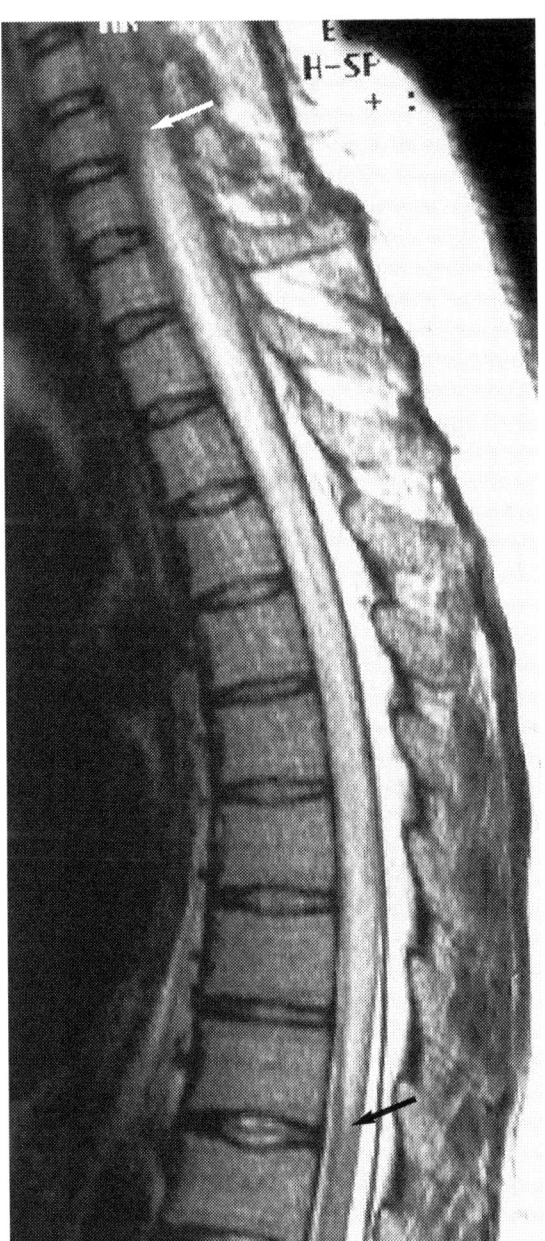

Figure 19. *This sagittal T2 WI demonstrates an extensive infarct of the spinal cord secondary to systemic hypotension. Note how the oedema associated with the infarction leads to a hyperintense signal on T2 WI.*

Epidural haematoma
On CT scans these lesions are hyperdense in the acute and subacute phases. On MR scanning the intensity varies according to the age of the lesion (see chapter 5). The location of the lesion in the extradural space helps with the diagnosis and it can be distinguished from an epidural abscess by the fact that it does not enhance with contrast and that there is no associated discitis or osteomyelitis.

6

CRANIAL AND SPINAL TUMOURS

Contents

Cranial tumours
Classification
Primary brain tumours
Metastatic tumours
Tumours at special sites

Spinal Tumours
Extradural compartment
Intradural, extramedullary compartment
Intramedullary compartment

Cranial tumours

Intracranial tumours account for about 2% of deaths from cancer. They may be primary, metastatic or extension from adjacent structures.

Classification

Primary intracranial tumours are classified according to the tissue of origin. (for the detailed WHO classification see the end of the chapter) A brief classification is as follows:

Primary brain tumours

1. Neuroepithelial tissue
   - Astrocytes — Astrocytoma
   - Oligodendrocytes — Oligodendroglioma
   - Ependyma — Ependymoma
   - Choroid plexus — Choroid plexus papilloma
   - Pineal gland — Pineocytoma, Pineoblastoma
   - Neuronal tissue — Gangliocytoma, ganglioglioma, neuroblastoma.
   - Empbryonic tissue — Glioblastoma, medulloblastoma

2. Nerve sheath cells
   - Neurilemmoma, neurofibroma

3. Meninges — Meningioma, melanoma

4.	Blood vessels	Haemangioblastoma
5.	Lymphatic tissue	Lymphoma
6.	Pituitary	Pituitary tumours
7.	Developmental malformations	Dermoid cysts, craniopharyngioma

Metastatic tumours

The brain is a common organ for metastases from several organs. Most common malignant tumours metastasise into the brain via the blood stream. However, distant spread to other organs of primary brain tumours is extremely rare.

Extension from Adjacent sites - tumours from adjacent structures in the base of skull such as carcinoma of the ethmoid sinuses, sphenoid sinuses and pharynx may grow upwards into the intracranial cavity and present with features of an intracranial tumour.

Pathophysiology

Different types of intracranial tumours have different effects on the brain. Tumours which are extra-cerebral (extra-axial) such as those arising from the pituitary gland, meninges, cranial nerves and the skull base tend to indent and displace the brain without destroying brain tissue. As such, they produce symptoms mainly as a result of neural compression. If such tumours are sufficiently large, they act as space occupying lesions leading to increased intracranial pressure. In contrast, tumours that grow within the brain parenchyma such as the neuroepithelial tumours, in addition to displacing also destroy brain tissue and produce symptoms from impaired function depending on the area involved. They also produce raised intracranial pressure (ICP) depending on the size. In addition, many brain tumours produce a reaction in the surrounding white matter leading to cerebral oedema that also contribute to the raised ICP.

Some tumours obstruct CSF pathways producing hydrocephalus that may result in raised ICP. Tumours such as those arising from the pituitary and the hypothalamus alter endocrine function leading to either hyper secretion or hypo secretion of hormones leading to different forms of endocrine disturbances.

Clinical presentation

Patients with brain tumours present with

a. Evidence of raised ICP
b. Focal neurological deficits
c. Epilepsy
d. Psychological disturbances
e. Endocrine disturbances
f. A combination of the above
g. Rarely tumours tend to bleed and present as spontaneous intra-cerebral haematoma

Raised ICP
Tumours that are sufficiently large act as space occupying lesions and produce raised ICP. The earliest features of raised ICP are headache, nausea, vomiting and papilloedema. The headache is usually continuous and worse in the mornings and accompanied by bouts of vomiting and nausea. It is aggravated by coughing and sneezing and tends to progressively increase in frequency and intensity as the tumour continues to enlarge. As the ICP increases, there is progressive impairment of consciousness recognized as a drop in GCS and with brain herniation, changes in vital signs and pupillary abnormalities that can eventually lead to death if untreated.

Focal neurological deficits
With neural compression and with destruction of neural tissue, function of the region involved begin to fail resulting in focal neurological deficits relevant to that area. These take the form of limb weakness, disturbances in sensation, gait, speech, and cranial nerve palsy. Focal neurological deficits provide a clinical indication of the site of the tumour.

Epilepsy
Brain tumours, especially those involving the cerebral hemispheres may cause epileptic seizures by altering the electrical activity of the surrounding brain. The seizures may be either focal or general. Epilepsy is most common in gliomas. meningiomas and metastases.

Psychological disturbances
Disturbances in behaviour may be the presenting feature in some of the brain tumours, specially those involving the frontal lobes. It is not uncommon for patients with long standing psychiatric illnesses to be subsequently diagnosed as having brain tumours.

Endocrine disturbances
Hormonal disturbances may occur due to hyper secretion of hormones by a tumour or hypo secretion due to destruction of functioning endocrine tissue by a tumour. Endocrine disturbances are common with pituitary tumours and hyper secretion may manifest as acromegaly, Cushing's syndrome, hyper prolactinaemia. Hypo secretion leads to hypo pituitarism. Pineal tumours also may cause hormonal disturbances manifesting as altered sexual function or pigmentation.

A combination of the above.
It is not uncommon for brain tumours to exhibit a combination of features listed above, depending on the site and size of the tumour. A large brain tumour may cause raised ICP and produce focal neurological deficits due to brain displacement or destruction and also lead to impaired consciousness that may manifest as abnormal behaviour.

Spontaneous intra-cerebral haematoma.
Rarely, brain tumours which are abnormally vascular may bleed spontaneously resulting in an intra cerebral haematoma or subarachnoid haemorrhage. The patient presents with a sudden event indicating a vascular pathology which on subsequent investigation proves to be haemorrhage from a tumour.

Investigations
Most brain tumours are evident with CT scanning. MRI provides more useful information regarding site, size, vascularity, relationship to surrounding structures and distribution of sur-

rounding brain oedema and the views may be reformatted to different planes so as to assist treatment planning. Angiography is useful if high vascularity is suspected.

Management

The different modalities of treatment for brain tumours include:

1. Surgical excision
2. Radiotherapy
3. Chemotherapy

Surgical excision
Excision of the tumour helps to arrive at a tissue diagnosis, restore normal ICP and relieve neural compression. The feasibility of total excision depends on the site of the tumour and its nature. Most of the benign tumours can be completely excised with minimal damage to the brain. However, malignant tumours that infiltrate the brain can only be treated with partial excision or biopsy if damage to functioning areas of the brain with consequent unacceptable neurological disability is to be avoided. Some of the benign tumours in relatively inaccessible positions are also treated with partial excision or biopsy.

Radiotherapy
External irradiation is useful in the management of some of the malignant tumours. Most malignant brain tumours carry a poor prognosis and although radiotherapy may delay recurrence of the tumour, complete cure is often not possible. Radiotherapy is also useful in preventing recurrence or controlling growth of some of the benign tumour that are treated with partial excision and complete cure could be achieved with rare tumours such as germinoma of the pineal gland. External radiation is applied to the whole brain, or focused to the area of the tumour. Stereotactic irradiation helps to focus accurately to small areas of tissue and can be achieved with a linear accelerator or with gamma rays.

Chemotherapy
Some of the malignant tumour are treated with anti mitotic agents which is usually used as adjuvent treatment to surgery and radiotherapy.

Prognosis

Benign tumours of the brain may be cured after total excision. However, there is a tendency to local recurrence in tumours such as meningiomas and pituitary adenomas. Malignant tumours tend to recur after removal despite treatment with radiotherapy and adjuvent methods. Some tumours such as glioblastomas have a very poor prognosis and most patients die within about an year or six months. However, metastases of brain tumours outside the nervous system are extremely rare.

Tumours at special sites

Certain tumours present with characteristic clinical features attributed to the site of the lesion e.g. pituitary tumours and cerebellopontine angle tumours.

Pituitary tumours

Tumours arising from the pituitary gland and its vicinity have characteristic clinical features due the anatomical proximity to various neural structures.

Surgical anatomy
The pituitary gland is contained within the sella turcica in the sphenoid bone and the floor of the pituitary fossa form part of the roof of the sphenoid sinus. Hence, enlargement of the pituitary fossa due to a tumour causes the pituitary fossa to bulge downwards into the sphenoid sinus. Hence, such lesions could be approached via the nasal cavity for surgical excision.

The optic chiasm, optic tracts and the optic nerves are positioned close to the roof of the pituitary fossa and tumours in this region (supra sellar tumours) as well as pituitary tumours enlarging upwards may cause pressure on these structures resulting in different visual field defects. Visual field defects are a common mode of presentation of pituitary tumours.

The cavernous sinus with the upper cranial nerves occupy the lateral aspects of the pituitary fossa and tumour enlarging laterally may cause multiple upper cranial nerve palsies.

The temporal lobes which are also placed laterally may be invaded by pituitary tumours leading to temporal lobe epilepsy.

Posteriorly, the pituitary fossa extends up to the clivus and dorsum sellae which is placed anterior to the interpeduncular fossa. Tumours growing backwards may grow into the interpeduncular fossa and cause compression of the cerebral peduncles leading to pyramidal signs in the extremities.

The third ventricle is situated superior to the pituitary fossa and upward extension of pituitary and supra sellar tumours may elevate the floor of the third ventricle and obstruct the foramina of Monro leading to hydrocephalus.

Pathophysiology and clinical features
Tumours arising from the pituitary gland as well as other supra sellar tumours such as meningiomas, optic nerve gliomas, giant anterior communicating artery aneurysms and craniopharyngiomas may compress the surrounding neural structures as indicated above resulting in different neurological deficits.

The common deficits are:

Optic chiasm	Bitemporal hemianopia
Optic tract	Homonymous hemianopia
Optic nerve	Unilateral blindness
Cavernous sinus	Palsy of IIIrd, IVth, VIth and ophthalmic div.Vth nerve
Third ventricle	Hydrocephalus and raised ICP
Interpeduncular fossa	Pyramidal signs
Sphenoid sinus	CSF rhinorrhoea

As the pituitary is an endocrine gland, tumours arising from cells that secrete different hormones (functioning tumours) may cause hyper secretion of certain hormones leading to different endocrine syndromes due to hormone excess such as acromegaly or gigantism, Cushin'gs syndrome and hyperprolactinaemia. Tumours that do not secrete hormones (non functioning tumours) may cause pressure on the normal pituitary gland leading to hypo secretion and hormone deficiency syndromes such as dwarfism, impaired sexual development and amenorrhoea.

Investigations

Plain X-rays of the skull may show enlargement of the pituitary fossa, erosion or calcification in the supra sellar region. CT scans may reveal large lesions and evidence of hydrocephalus. More accurate visualisation of the extent in different directions is possible with MRI. Angiography is carried out if an aneurysm is suspected.

Management

The aims of management are relief of neural compression especially the optic pathways that if untreated could result in blindness, extirpation of as much tumour as possible and prevention of recurrence and management of hormonal disturbances. These aims are achieved with surgical means, radiotherapy or a combination of both. Surgical excision is carried out via the nasal passages (trans sphenoidal excision) where the tumour enlarges the pituitary fossa downwards into the sphenoid sinus or via a craniotomy (sub frontal approach) where the tumour extends mainly upwards (supra sellar extension). Hormonal disturbances require monitoring of blood levels and replacement of hormones where appropriate.

Cerebellopontine angle tumours

Tumours arising in the region of the cerebellopontine angle (C-P angle) may cause compression of the cerebellum, pons, fourth ventricle or lower cranial nerves resulting in characteristic clinical features.

Surgical anatomy

The C-P angle is located deep to the mastoid process and is an area bounded by the cerebellum and pons medially, the petrous bone laterally and containing the lower cranial nerves Vth, VIth, VIIth, VIIIth, IXth, Xth, XIth and XIIth nerves. The fourth ventricle opens into the C-P angle cistern via the foramen of Luschka. The vertebral artery and its branches such as the posterior inferior cerebellar arteries as well as the superior cerebellar arteries are also contained within the C-P angle.

Pathophysiology

The common tumours within the C-P angle are Schwanomas such as acoustic neuroma (vestibular schwannoma), meningiomas and cholesteotoma or epidermoid cyst (a non neoplastic lesion). As these lesions enlarge, they cause pressure on the various cranial nerves resulting in corresponding cranial nerve palsy. Enlargement towards the cerebellum may results in disturbance of cerebellar function. Enlargement towards the pons may cause pyramidal signs in the extremities. Displacement and obstruction of the 4th ventricle may result in hydrocephalus and features of raised ICP.

Clinical presentation

Patients with C-P angle tumours present with features referable to the different structures involved in the lesion as follows:

Cerebellum	Cerebellar signs, ataxia, vertigo, clumsiness, nystagmus.
Pons	Pyramidal signs, spasticity
Vth nerve	Sensory symptoms in face, wasting & weakness of masseters, pterygoids & temporalis
VIth nerve	Diplopia, VIth nerve palsy
VIIth nerve	Lower motor neuron facial palsy of ipsilateral side

VIIIth nerve	(Cochlear)	Tinnitus deafness
	(Vestibular)	Vertigo, loss of balance
IXth nerve		Nasal regurgitation, absence of gag
Xth nerve		Palatal palsy, hoarseness of voice, nasal regurgitation
XIth nerve		Weakness of trapezius, sternomastoid
XIIth nerve		Wasting and weakness of tongue
Fourth ventricle		Hydrocephalus and raised ICP, headache, vomiting & papilloedema

Investigation

Most C-P angle lesions are demonstrated by CT & MRI scanning.

Management

As most C-P angle tumours are benign, surgical excision with prospect of cure is possible in most instances. The current use of the operating microscope has greatly improved the surgical results in terms of morbidity and mortality by avoiding per-operative damage to cranial nerves, important blood vessels and the pons.

Spinal Tumours

Tumours of the spine are located in one of three anatomical compartments, the extradural compartment, the intradural, extramedullary compartment or the intramedullary compartment.

Extradural compartment

Primary tumours

Bony tumours
Osteoid osteoma

This is a benign skeletal neoplasm presenting in young people but rarely in children younger than five. The salient clinical feature is pain that is worse at night and is relieved by small doses of salicylates. On imaging, the lesion presents as a small island of sclerotic bone with a radiolucent centre that is usually less than 1.5 cm in diameter. Radionuclide scans are a good way to locate the tumours. The tumour sometimes involutes spontaneously. Treatment is with surgical excision or radiofrequency ablation and the aim is complete ablation or resection of the tumour, which is curative.

Osteoblastoma

This is a benign tumour that is closely related to the osteoid osteoma and is differentiated by the ability of the nidus to grow larger than two centimeters. Patients usually present in the first three decades of life. It has to be differentiated from the aggressive osteosarcoma. On imaging, the lesion usually presents as a well-circumscribed radiolucent lesion with a thin rim of new bone that separates it from the surrounding soft tissues. Osteoblastomas that are more aggressive display local resorption of the cortex, destruction of bone, and extension into surrounding soft tissues. For tumours that remain subcapsular local resection is acceptable. More aggressive types with extracapsular extension require resection with a wide margin, which is usually curative.

Osteosarcoma

This malignant tumour usually presents in the lumbosacral spine in the fourth decade of life and has a male preponderance. These tumours present with pain and local mass effects. On imaging, this is usually a tumour of the vertebral body that extends into the soft tissues and may incorporate the posterior elements. The tumour is usually intensely hyperdense and the vertebrae have been called ivory vertebrae. There is frequently a loss of height of the vertebrae. Despite wide surgical resection and adjuvant chemotherapy and radiotherapy, the diagnosis is poor with life expectancy usually less than two years.

Cartilaginous tumours of the spine
Osteochondroma

These are benign tumours presenting in the third and fourth decades of life. They involve the cervical spine mostly (especially C2) and are usually located in the posterior elements. On imaging the lesion presents as an exostosis with a cartilaginous cap. In adults this cap should be less than 2 cm, if not; malignant transformation to chondrosarcoma should be suspected. Complete surgical resection is usually curative.

Chondrosarcoma

These are malignant tumours presenting mostly in men in the fifth decade of life and most commonly in the thoracic spine. They present on imaging with a characteristic matrix arranged in the form of rings and arcs and in approximately 30% extend through the disc spaces into adjacent levels. Complete cure can be achieved with total excision and a wide margin. Adjuvant chemotherapy may be used to reduced tumour mass. These lesions have the potential to metastasise (mostly to the lungs) and lesions that are not resected with a wide margin mostly recur.

Lymphoproliferative tumours
Multiple myeloma

This is a systemic disease of middle-aged people caused by malignant plasma cells that produce elevated levels of immunoglobulins. This is the most common primary bone tumour and presents with local bone destruction. Diagnosis is confirmed by detecting immunoglobulins with protein electrophoresis in the patient's serum and urine. The mainstay of treatment is radiation therapy and chemotherapy with surgical stabilisation of destructed and unstable levels.

Solitary plasmacytoma

These are also caused by malignant plasma cells, but are solitary lesions that occur in younger people and have a better prognosis. Radiation therapy and surgical stabilisation as above are the mainstay of treatment. These lesions can transform into multiple myeloma and it is important to follow patients up life long.

Lymphoma

This can either be primary lymphoma of the bone or secondary deposits of both Hodgkin and non-Hodgkin lymphomas (cranial lymphoma is Non-Hodgkin). These patients present with local compressive effects due to tumour growth. On imaging lymphoma appears as a large soft tissue mass extending from the bone and is homogenous and hypointense on T1 WI images and enhances strongly with contrast. Technetium bone scans are very sensitive in detecting these lesions. The mainstay of treatment is radiotherapy with surgery reserved for cases requiring decompression and stabilisation.

Tumours of notochordal origin
Chordoma
These tumours arise from a notochord remnant (the notochord evolves into the nucleus pulposus of the intervertebral discs). These are large soft tissue masses and have associated vertebral destruction. More than half demonstrate calcification on imaging and they are hypointense on T1 WI and hyperintense on T2 WI since they have high water content and enhance with contrast administration. Surgical resection with adjuvant chemotherapy and radiotherapy is the treatment of choice. Sacrococcygeal tumours have 8-10 year survival and tumours at other sites have 4-5 year survival. These lesions may metastasise but death is usually due to the local effects of the tumour.

Round cell tumours
Ewing sarcoma
These malignant tumours occur in children and mostly in the sacrococcygeal region. Diffuse sclerosis is usually evident on imaging and these lesions are usually located in the vertebral bodies with soft tissue extension. Treatment consists of radiotherapy and chemotherapy and this achieves nearly 100% local control with nearly 90% long-term survival. This is less true for sacral tumours since they are usually larger at presentation.

Metastatic tumours
The tumours that most commonly metastasise to the spine are carcinoma of the prostate, breast adenocarcinoma, lung adenocarcinoma, renal cell carcinoma and gastric carcinoma. Treatment is based on several factors including the general status of the patient, status of the systemic disease, amount of neural compression and the presence of intractable pain. Metastatic tumours cannot be cured by local excision of the metastasis and the treatment is aimed at local decompression of the tumour. Concurrent stability procedures are aimed at preserving anatomical integrity and for pain relief. The mainstay of treatment for metastatic tumours of the spine is radiotherapy.

Intradural, extramedullary compartment

Nerve sheath tumours
Neurofibromas and schwannomas are derived from a common Schwann cell origin. Neurofibromas are made up of fibrous tissues as well as nerve fibres. In neurofibromas there is a fusiform enlargement of the nerve and it is not possible to distinguish between the nerve tissue and the fibrous tissue. Schwannomas are round or ovoid masses that are suspended from the nerve and are made up of bipolar cells that are either arranged in a palisade formation, called Antoni – A or are loosely arranged, called Antoni – B. The latter is less common. These tumours occur between the fourth and the sixth decade, arise mostly from a dorsal nerve root, and are mostly intradural. Some extend through a neural foramen as the classical dumbbell tumours and rarely they are entirely extradural. These are benign tumours and the treatment is excision with excellent prognosis.

Meningiomas
Both these and the nerve sheath tumours make up 25% each of intradural tumours. They arise from the arachnoid cap cells on the dura at the edge of the root sleeve and are therefore found mostly in a lateral position. There is a female preponderance and they arise mostly in the thoracic spine. These are also mostly benign lesions, just like their cranial counterparts and treatment is complete excision with excellent prognosis.

Filum terminale ependymomas
Nearly half of spinal canal ependymomas arise in the filum terminale. There is a slight male preponderance and these tumours tend to occur in the third to fifth decade of life. The histological arrangement is myxopapillary and consists of tumour cells surrounding a core of hyalinised and poorly differentiated connective tissue. These are benign tumours for the most part and the treatment is excision.

Intramedullary compartment

Ependymoma (55% of intramedullary tumours)
These benign tumours occur mostly in men in the fourth decade. They can occur throughout out the spine but a specific type, the myxopapillary ependymoma arises in the conus and filum terminale. These tumours are homogenous and well circumscribed, discrete and cause their symptoms by intrinsic compression of the spinal cord rather than infiltration. They are hypointense on T1 WI, enhance strongly with contrast and are hyperintense on T2 WI. Resection results in prolonged survival. Some lesions may undergo malignant transformation, infiltrate, and metastasise within the CNS.

Astrocytoma (30% of intramedullary tumours)
Low-grade astrocytomas and pilocytic astrocytomas are slow growing, usually have cleavage planes and may be totally or nearly totally excised. Residual tumours may be treated expectantly although the treatment of these residual tumours is controversial. Anaplastic glioma and glioblastoma multiforme are rare but lethal. Resection of these malignant tumours is not possible and life expectancy is generally less than 2 years.

Other tumours
Generally these tumours have the same imaging characteristics of their cranial counter parts. Intramedullary oligodendrogliomas are rare, the optimal management is not yet known and chemotherapy sensitivity, unlike the cranial type, is unproven. Dermoid cysts, epidermoid cysts and lipomas are inclusion tumours that are slow growing. The aim of treatment is total resection with prolonged survival in dermoid cysts and epidermoid cysts but lipomas are frequently difficult to excise completely. Hemangioblastomas can be cured by complete removal. They are vascular and piecemeal removal is risky. Gangliogliomas are more common in childhood, are benign and the aim of treatment is total resection with prolonged survival. Subependymoma are rare lesions and experience with their management is limited but total resection is the main aim of treatment.

WHO classification of CNS tumours

Neuroepithelial tumours of the CNS

Gliomas
Astrocytic tumours
(Low grade) Astrocytoma (WHO grade II)
Anaplastic (malignant) astrocytoma (WHO grade III)
Glioblastoma multiforme (WHO grade IV)
Pilocytic astrocytoma [non-invasive, WHO grade I]
Subependymal giant cell astrocytoma (non-invasive, WHO grade I)
Pleomorphic xanthoastrocytoma (non-invasive, WHO grade I)

Oligodendroglial tumours
Oligodendroglioma (WHO grade II)
Anaplastic (malignant) oligodendroglioma (WHO grade III)

Ependymal cell tumours
Ependymoma (WHO grade II)
Anaplastic ependymoma (WHO grade III)
Myxopapillary ependymoma
Subependymoma (WHO grade I)

Mixed gliomas
Mixed oligoastrocytoma (WHO grade II)
Anaplastic (malignant) oligoastrocytoma (WHO grade III)

Neuroepithelial tumours of uncertain origin
Polar spongioblastoma (WHO grade IV)
Astroblastoma (WHO grade IV)
Gliomatosis cerebri (WHO grade IV)

Tumours of the choroid plexus
Choroid plexus papilloma
Choroid plexus carcinoma (anaplastic choroid plexus papilloma)

Neuronal and mixed neuronal-glial tumours
Gangliocytoma
Dysplastic gangliocytoma of cerebellum (Lhermitte-Duclos)
Ganglioglioma
Anaplastic (malignant) ganglioglioma
Desmoplastic infantile ganglioglioma
Central neurocytoma
Dysembryoplastic neuroepithelial tumor
Olfactory neuroblastoma (esthesioneuroblastoma)

Pineal parenchymal tumours
Pineocytoma
Pineoblastoma

Mixed pineocytoma/pineoblastoma

Tumours with neuroblastic or glioblast elements (embryonal tumours)
Medulloepithelioma
Primitive neuroectodermal tumours with multipotent differentiation
Medulloblastoma
Cerebral primitive neuroectodermal tumor
Neuroblastoma
Retinoblastoma
Ependymoblastoma

Other CNS Neoplasms

Tumours of the sellar region
Pituitary adenoma
Pituitary carcinoma
Craniopharyngioma

Hematopoietic tumours
Primary malignant lymphomas
Plasmacytoma
Granulocytic sarcoma

Germ cell tumours
Germinoma
Embryonal carcinoma
Yolk sac tumor (endodermal sinus tumor)
Choriocarcinoma
Teratoma
Mixed germ cell tumours

Tumours of the meninges
Meningioma
Atypical meningioma
Anaplastic (malignant) meningioma
Non-meningothelial tumours of the meninges

Benign mesenchymal tumours
Osteocartilaginous tumours
Lipoma
Fibrous histiocytoma

Malignant mesenchymal tumours
Chondrosarcoma
Haemangiopericytoma
Rhabdomyosarcoma
Meningeal sarcomatosis

Primary melanocytic lesions
Diffuse melanosis
Melanocytoma
Malignant melanoma

Tumours of uncertain histogenesis
Hemangioblastoma

Tumours of cranial and spinal nerves
Schwannoma (neurinoma, neurilemoma)
Neurofibroma
Malignant peripheral nerve sheath tumor (Malignant schwannoma)

Local extensions from regional tumours
Paraganglioma (chemodectoma)
Chordoma
Chondrosarcoma
Carcinoma

Metastatic tumours

Unclassified tumours

Cysts and tumour-like lesions
Rathke cleft cyst
Epidermoid
Dermoid
Colloid cyst of the third ventricle
Enterogenous cyst
Neuroglial cyst
Granular cell tumour (choristoma, pituicytoma)
Hypothalamic neuronal hamartoma
Nasal glial herterotopia
Plasma cell granuloma

7

VASCULAR ABNORMALITIES

Contents

Intracranial vascular abnormalities
   Arteriovenous malformations (AVM)
   Cavernous angiomas
   Venous angiomas
   Cerebral aneurysms
Spontaneous subarachnoid heamorrhage (SAH)

Intracranial vascular abnormalities

The intracranial vasculature develops pathology in several ways. There may be occlusion of arteries or venous structures or haemorrhage can occur into the parenchyma, the intraventricular system, the subdural space or subarachnoid space.

Occlusion of cerebral blood vessels is usually due to embolic phenomena and these can be secondary to atherosclerotic plaques, infected emboli or foreign material. Occlusion of the arterial side of the circulation leads to ischaemia and, if the blood flow is not restored instantly, it will lead to cell death and infarction. Occlusion of the venous part of the circulation will lead to venous hypertension, intraparenchymal bleeds and infarction. Hypertensive spontaneous intraparenchymal bleeds are secondary to the rupture of friable blood vessels. Spontaneous haemorrhages can also be secondary to vascular anomalies and/or aneurysms.

Arteriovenous malformations (AVM) are lesions in which the arterial system short-circuits directly into the venous system without the intervening capillary bed. The venous circulation is not designed to function under such high pressure and this leads to tortuous vessels and associated flow aneurysms may also develop. AVM's recruit additional blood vessels and may grow quite large. They are graded according to the Spetzler-Martin grading scale based on three factors, namely the size of the lesion, its location and the type of venous drainage. AVM's either cause effects secondarily to brain irritation (seizures) or may present with spontaneous intraparenchymal bleeds.

Cavernous angiomas (cavernomas, cavernous malformations) do not fill from the systemic circulation and do not drain via veins but rather are abnormal thin-walled vascular channels (caverns). They can present with spontaneous haemorrhage or seizures and are more prevalent in the paediatric population. Cavernous angiomas are sometimes found in the spinal cord and can cause potentially devastating neurological sequelae secondary to haemorrhage.

Size	Score	Eloquent brain	Score	Deep draining vein	Score
more than 6cm	3	Yes	1	Yes	1
3-6cm	2	No	0	No	0
less than 3cm	1				

Table 1. *The Spetzler-Martin grading scale. The size of the lesion is divided into categories of less than 3cms (1 point), 3-6cms (2 points) and greater than 6cms (3 points). If the AVM is located in an eloquent area of the brain such as the speech area, motor area, visual cortex or brain stem then another point is added. If the venous draining system is deep and if the lesion, for instance, drains directly into the vein of Galen or the straight sinus, then another point is added. The maximum score therefore is five.*

Since cavernomas do not fill or drain from the systemic circulation, they are diagnosed on MRI scanning and are non-detectable on angiography. Lesions can be watched expectantly if they are discovered incidentally. Symptomatic lesions with multiple haemorrhagic events, can be treated surgically if accessible, or with radio surgery if surgically inaccessible.

Venous angiomas are most likely to have formed during the embryonic period due to an arrest of venous development. They are composed of dilated venous channels that drain normal brain and converge into medullary veins which are enlarged and these in turn drain into normal cortical veins. They may sometimes be found in association with cavernous angiomas. The majority of these lesions are discovered incidentally and present only infrequently with haemorrhage. These lesions can be diagnosed on MRI scanning as well as angiography. On contrasted MRI scanning they form a characteristic 'caput medusa lesion' where dilated capillary veins drain centrally towards a main draining vein. They can be diagnosed on angiography when, in the venous phase, a persistent pattern of dilated medullary veins is seen that drains towards a single draining vein. They are usually managed expectantly.

Cerebral aneurysms are usually found amongst the medium sized arteries of the circle of Willis and can be fusiform dilatations or saccular berry aneurysms. Saccular aneurysms form due to weakness of the interna and media of the artery wall resulting in outpouching. These are true aneurysms. False aneurysms can be found secondary to trauma or infection and are not contained by the vessel wall but rather by the surrounding tissues. Aneurysms are thought to be flow related in their mechanism of origin and are usually found at vessel bifurcation on the side of the greatest flow.

Some inherited conditions are associated with the formation of cerebral aneurysms, including polycystic kidney disease, Ehlers-Danlos syndrome, Marfan syndrome and neurofibromatosis type 1. Aneurysms, unlike the other malformations noted above, usually present with subarachnoid haemorrhage as they are located in the subarachnoid space. The other lesions usually cause intraparenchymal haemorrhage. In cases of intraparenchymal haemorrhage, the clinical effects are due to direct destruction of brain and to secondary pressure effects of the intraparenchymal clot. In the case of aneurysms that have previously leaked, the dome of the aneurysm can become adherent to brain and subsequent bleeds can also have an intraparenchymal component. Saccular (berry) aneurysms are classified according to size into small (less than 10mm), large (more than 10mm) and giant (greater than 25mm); their location in the anterior or posterior circulation of the circle of Willis and which blood vessel they originate from. The risk of rupture grows with increase in size and rupture usually occurs when the aneurysm reaches 5-10mm. Rupture commonly occurs during activities that increase blood pressure and a constant environmental factor that has been associated with increased risk of subarachnoid haemorrhage is cigarette smoking.

Spontaneous subarachnoid heamorrhage (SAH)

Spontaneous subarachnoid heamorrhage (SAH) is a common neurosurgical emergency and accounts for 5% of all strokes. In the UK the incidence of SAH is 10/100,000 population per year. the incidence varies geographically and is about 5 - 15 /100,000 in western European USA, 3.5 in South Africa, and 25 in Japan. In UK, about 5000 to 6000 cases are admitted each year and in USA about 28000. The sex ratio is M : F is 1 : 1.5 and the common age of presentation is 40 - 60 years.

The common causes of spontaneous SAH are:

1. Abnormalities in intracranial blood vessels
    Aneurysms 70 -75%
    Arterio venous malformations (AVMs) 5%
    Moya Moya disease, seen mostly in Japan
2. Abnormalities in blood with bleeding tendency
    Haemophilias
    Other coagulopathies
    Anticoagulant treatment (Eg. warfarin)
    Antiplatelet treatment (Eg. aspirin)
3. Generalised diseases predisposing to haemorrhage
    Hypertension
    Vasculitis
    Collagen disorders such as lupus
4. Intracranial tumours

Spontaneous SAH from ruptured aneurysms is the commonest. Among those with ruptured aneurysms, 15% die before admission to hospital, after admission to hospital, if untreated, 15%, die within the first 24 hours, 15% within 1 day to 2 weeks, 15% from 2 weeks to 2 months and 15% from 2 months to 2 years and about 10% per year thereafter. Even after treatment, the mortality is still high and 6% die from re-bleeding and 7% from vasospasm. 1% of those who survive re-bleeding and 7% of those who survive vasospasm are left severely disabled. The majority of aneurysms occur around the circle of Willis and 90% are in relation to the anterior circulation while 10% are in the posterior circulation.

Pathophysiology
Aneurysms form due to a weakness of the vessel wall usually at a point of branching where there is a defect in the media of the vessel wall. The tendency to form aneurysms may be hereditary and sometimes there is also a familial incidence. The bulging vessel wall distends to a sac which eventually ruptures. Sometimes the sac can be enormous and result in pressure on adjacent neural structures such as the optic chiasm or nerve or other cranial nerves

such as the third or sixth. At the point of rupture of an aneurysm, the rush of arterial blood into the intracranial cavity causes a sudden increase of ICP to nearly systolic blood pressure. This could cause immediate damage to surrounding brain tissue as well as a massive autonomic disturbance that could result in a cardiac arrest. However, the majority of patients survive this episode and get admitted to hospital. The blood in the subarachnoid space causes meningeal irritation leading to photophobia and neck stiffness. Sometimes there could be concomitant haemorrhage into the brain parenchyma causing an intra-cerebral haematoma (ICH) that could result in focal brain damage as well as raised ICP if the ICH is sufficiently large.

Following the initial haemorrhage, very often the point of rupture of the aneurysm is sealed with a thrombus. The presence of blood in the CSF activates a chemical reaction due to degradation of the blood resulting in build up of fibrinolytic enzymes in the CSF. This build up reaches a peak around the 7th to 14th day and is responsible for lysis of the thrombus that had earlier sealed the point of rupture. This results in re-bleeding and on this occasion thrombus formation is impaired due to the fibrinolytic activity in the CSF and very often re-bleeding proves to be fatal.

The presence of degraded blood products in the CSF also contributes to accumulation of chemicals responsible for vasospasm and this results in varying degrees of spasm of main arteries that will eventually cause ischaemia and infarction of brain tissue.
The blood pigment in CSF also damages the arachnoid granulations resulting in poor CSF absorption leading to a communicating hydrocephalus. Hydrocephalus could also be caused by obstruction to CSF flow from intra-ventricular blood clots.

Complications of aneurysmal rupture
Intracranial
1. Damage to neural tissue at point of haemorrahge due to sudden rise of ICP
2. Focal brain damage from intracerebral haemorrhage (ICH)
3. Raised ICP from ICH
4. Re-bleeding
5. Vasospasm and cerebral ischaemia and infarction
6. Hydrocephalus
5. Epilepsy

Extra cranial (mainly due to autonomic dysfunction)
1. Cardiac arrhythmias
2. Myocardial infarction
3. Pulmonary oedema
4. Gastric haemorrhage
5. Hypo or hypertension

Patients with spontaneous SAH present with sudden onset of very severe headache. The onset is so sudden that patients often recall what exactly they were doing when they were struck down by the headache. Often the headache is accompanied by nausea and vomiting and they may lose consciousness. Due to the presence of blood in the subarachnoid space, they have signs of meningeal irritation such as photophobia, neck stiffness and a positive Kernig's sign. Sometimes, they also develop a focal neurological deficit with the onset of the headache.

Depending on the extent of brain damage the clinical picture of the patient on admission could vary in severity and has been classified to different clinical grades. The World Federation of Neurological Surgeons (WFNS) suggested the following grades which also seem to correlate with outcome. The WFNS grade which is now used widely is based on the GCS score and is as follows:

WFNS Grade	GCS score	Motor deficit
I	15	None
II	14 - 13	none
III	14 - 13	present
IV	12 - 7	present or absent
V	6 - 3	present or absent

Patients admitted with the above history should have an immediate CT scan which often shows the blood in the subarachnoid space and the basal cisterns. In cases where there is a good history but negative CT scan, lumbar puncture and spectroscopy is invaluable. Following SAH, the red blood cells that entered the CSF undergo lysis and it takes several hours for the liberated oxyhaemoglobin to be converted via deoxyhaemoglobin to bilirubin. The enzyme, haem-oxygenase, which is responsible for the process is only found in the CNS. If a period of 12 hours is allowed following a suspected SAH, CSF obtained with a lumbar puncture can be spun down and spectroscopy performed on it. The presence of bilirubin is diagnostic for SAH. This is a very sensitive test for the first 14 days following SAH. The test should be delayed for 12 hours to allow the break down process into bilirubin to be completed, if not, a traumatic tap will be too early to pick up bilirubin and may contaminate the CSF sufficiently to make future test unreliable. The presence of high systemic levels of bilirubin and high levels of CNS protein may give false positive results but there are formulae to compensate for this. Those patients in poor clinical grades are first resuscitated and their cardiovascular state restored with medical means. Angiography is deferred until they improve to a better grade. If there is an immediate threat to life by raised ICP due to an ICH, this has to be removed as an emergency.

Specific effects of SAH

The medical management of SAH is extremely important and is based on the prevention of rebleeding and symptomatic vasospasm. The greatest risk of rebleeding is on the first day (4.1%) and the cumulative risk in the first two weeks is 19%. Rebleeding is associated with a 78% mortality rate and strict bed rest, restriction of visitors, quiet surroundings, adequate analgesia, stool softeners and antihypertensive agents when the mean arterial pressure (MAP) exceeds 130 mm Hg are measures used to try to prevent this catastrophe. Intravenous beta-blockers are popular for blood pressure control since they have a relatively short half-life, can be titrated easily and do not increase ICP. Seizures occur in as many as 25% of patients following SAH (most common in middle cerebral artery aneurysms) and increase the risk of rebleeding. Two anticonvulsants that allow for rapid IV loading, Phenytoin and Phenobarbital, are both used for prophylaxis. Patients in a poor grade and with increased ICP should be intubated and ventilated and care taken to keep the pCO_2 between 30-35 mm Hg (4-4.6 kPa), avoiding excessive hyperventilation which may cause vasospasm and brain ischaemia/infarction. The cerebral perfusion pressure (CPP) should be kept above 60-70 mm Hg.

Vasospasm
Vasospasm mostly occurs 4-14 days after the haemorrhage and is present in up to 70% of patients. Clinically symptomatic vasospasm is present in up to 30% of patients, may lead to cerebral ischaemia and infarction, and is more common in females, young patients, those who smoke, patients who presents in a poor clinical grade and those with large volumes of blood in the subarachnoid space. Patients present with a new onset decrease in consciousness or focal neurological deficit. Conventional angiography is the gold standard for diagnosing vasospasm but the diagnosis can be made reliably as a bedside test with transcranial Doppler. Other imaging modalities including single photon emission computed tomography (SPECT) and perfusion imaging (Xenon CT, dynamic perfusion CT and MRI), have been used successfully.

Prophylaxis for vasospasm:
Prophylaxis with Nimodipine is now standard practice and it improves overall outcome within 3 months of aneurysmal SAH. It appears that Nimodipine may have a neuroprotective effect by blocking calcium influx into damaged brain cells. Current practice is to maintain normovolemia to slight hypervolemia to prevent hypoperfusion. Results suggest that subarachnoid blood removal with intracisternal injections of recombinant tissue plasminogen activator (rTPA) during surgery for aneurysm clipping may carry some benefit.

Treatment for proven vasospasm:
Hypertensive, hypervolemic, and haemodilution therapy (HHH therapy, triple H), the standard of treatment for proven vasospasm, should be reserved for patients with secured aneurysms to reduce the risk of rebleeding.
Hypervolemia - The central venous pressure (CVP) should be maintained at 10-12 mm Hg. The pulmonary artery wedge pressure (PAWP) should be maintained at 19-20 mm Hg.
Haemodilution - The hematocrit should be maintained at 30-35% with dilution or packed cell transfusion to optimise blood viscosity and oxygen delivery.
Hypertensive therapy - Inotropic support and vasopressors may be needed to keep the mean arterial pressure (MAP) between 90 and 110 mm Hg.
Cerebral angiography with transluminal balloon angioplasty has been reported to lead to improved neurologic outcome in 70% of patients with symptomatic vasospasm. It is effective in treatment of large proximal vessels and is not effective in treatment of smaller distal vessels. Cerebral angiography with intra-arterial injection of Papaverine and nimodipine is also effective. Approximately 15-20% of patients with symptomatic vasospasm will have a poor outcome despite maximal therapy.

Definitive treatment of the aneurysm
Both surgical clipping and endovascular obliteration are highly successful treatments modalities. The international subarachnoid aneurysm trial (ISAT) which included mostly patients with small anterior circulation aneurysms showed a 22.5% relative and 6.9% absolute risk reduction at one year in the disability outcome of patients who were treated with coiling compared to those treated with surgery. There are many caveats to the interpretation of this study and the results cannot be extrapolated to all aneurysms. It has however fixed endovascular management firmly in the mind of physicians and the lay public alike. The main concern of endovascular treatment is the paucity of data on the longevity of this form of treatment. The following are broad guidelines:

Indications for surgical clipping include
Presence of a large parenchymal haematoma that requires evacuation
Young, fit patients with a good clinical grade (WFNS or Hunt and Hess grades 1-3)
Giant aneurysms
Complicated vascular anatomy with arteries originating from the aneurysmal dome
Wide-necked aneurysms (the coils escape from the aneurysm and block distal vessels)
Recurrent aneurysm after endovascular treatment with coil embolisation
Patient's wishes

Indications for endovascular treatment include
Patients who are medically unfit for a long general anaesthetic
Patients presenting with a poor clinical grade
Aneurysms located in the cavernous sinus and basilar tip aneurysm
Patients with symptomatic vasospasm who may benefit from endovascular treatment of their vasospasm
Multiple aneurysms not located close together anatomically
Patient's wishes

Timing of the intervention
Early surgery within the first 3 days allows for the prevention of rebleeding, the removal of blood clots that may reduce vasospasm and for the use of maximal HHH therapy since transluminal pressure fluctuations are negated by clipping. However surgery is technically more difficult due to brain swelling and fragility of the aneurysm dome with increased surgical morbidity. Delayed surgery removes most of the technical difficulties except for very late surgery that brings the complication of adhesions. However, the aneurysm remains unprotected for this period and rebleeding carries a high mortality rate. It has been found that patients with good grades (grade 1 and 2) fare better with early treatment. This is less conclusive for grade 3 patients and grade 4 and 5 patients should be managed on a case per case basis. Patients with significant hydrocephalus may sometimes improve significantly on their clinical grading with the simple act of placing an external ventricular drain (EVD). Many centres employ endovascular treatment as a first line of management for patients in a poor clinical grade and some centres are using endovascular treatment as the mainstay of treatment.

Management of ruptured AVMs
Ruptured AVMs frequently cause intra-cerebral heamorrhage with or without SAH. The incidence of complications such as re-bleeding and vasospasm are less than that for aneurysm. The aim of treatment is to prevent re-bleeding and if possible excise or thrombose the AVM. This can be achieved surgically where the AVM is in an accessible non eloquent area of the brain. Other forms of treatment are endovascular embolisaton and radiosurgery where gamma rays or X-rays from a linear accelerator are focused to the AVM after stereotactic localization resulting in slow thrombosis of the nidus. This is especially useful with AVMs in surgically inaccessible areas and where endovascular treatment carries a high risk of extension of thrombosis and infarction of eloquent areas of the brain.

8

CEREBRAL INFARCTION AND HAEMORRHAGE

Contents

Cerebral haemorrhage
Cerebral infarction

Cerebral infarction and haemorrhage are common cerebro-vascular accidents which present as a sudden onset of a neurological deficit with or without loss of consciousness. Loss of consciousness is more common with cerebral haemorrhage than with infarction.

Cerebral haemorrhage

Spontaneous haemorrhage into the brain parenchyma (intra cerebral haemorrhage or ICH) occurs when a blood vessel usually under arterial pressure ruptures into the brain substance. This could occur due a variety of reasons which are similar to those causing spontaneous sub-arachnoid haemorrhage (SAH). Indeed, it is not uncommon for spontaneous SAH to co-exist with ICH.

Pathophysiology
When a blood vessel under arterial pressure ruptures into the brain substance, the strong jet of blood cuts through the soft brain with an acute increase in intracranial pressure. This acute rise in ICP could result in immediate loss of consciousness. The point of rupture is usually sealed with a thrombus and the extravasated blood collects in a pool within the brain parenchyma. The pool of blood soon coagulates to form a solid blood clot.
The subsequent clinical picture depends on the size of the blood clot and the location. If the blood clot is relatively small, there could be sufficient compensation within the intracranial cavity so that any mass effect is minimal. However, if the clot is of a sufficiently large size, it acts as a space occupying lesion and causes increased ICP and brain displacement. Raised ICP could also be caused by an ICH blocking CSF pathways such in the cerebellum resulting in obstructive hydrocephalus.
Following the initial haematoma formation, there is commonly secondary change in the damaged brain parenchyma due to various chemicals that are released in the region of the ICH. These result in a degree of cerebral oedema that would further contribute to the raised ICP and also extend the area of brain damage beyond the confines of the original ICH.
Depending on the location of the clot, there could be focal neurological deficits. The damage done to the brain when the jet of blood cuts through would result in disruption of white

matter pathways leading to loss of function in the relevant areas. The common deficits are hemiparesis, cerebellar signs and multiple cranial nerve palsy in case of brain stem ICH. If the ICH occupies a 'silent' area of the brain, there would be no focal neurological deficit.

Clinical features
Patients with spontaneous ICH present with a sudden onset of a neurological deficit with or without loss of consciousness. There is frequently accompanying headache. Changes in GCS score, size of the pupils and vital signs may be present depending on the extent of raised ICP caused by the ICH. CT scans show the site and extent of the ICH as well as complications such as hydrocephalus or accompanying oedema.

Management
The management is directed towards identifying a cause for the haemorrhage and treating the ICH.
Identification of the cause of the haemorrhage involves estimation INR and investigation of other clotting abnormalities as well identifying systemic hypertension and appropriate management. In the absence of a systemic cause, angiography is used to identify any local abnormality of blood vessels.
If the ICH is of a sufficiently large size and causing raised intracranial pressure, it has to be evacuated as an emergency to prevent irreversible brain damage due to uncontrolled ICP. If the ICH is relatively small, it would re-absorb with time and treatment is directed towards the cause of the haemorrhage and prevention of future recurrence depending on the cause. This is achieved by surgical, endovascular or radiosurgical means or a combination of these modalities.

Cerebral infarction
Cerebral infarction occurs when a blood vessel to a certain part of the brain is blocked.

Pathophysiology
Blood vessels in the brain could be blocked as a result of local thrombus formation on an atheromatous plaque or due to an embolus of distant origin. Blocking of a blood vessel proximal to the circle of Willis could be compensated to some extent depending on the integrity of the circle but the vessels beyond have minimal cross anastomoses and behave as end vessels. Obstruction to such an artery results in ischaemia in the area of supply of that artery which could lead to infarction.
There is a physiological reserve in the requirements of perfusion of brain tissue and certain degrees of cerebral ischaemia could be compensated without any evidence of cerebral dysfunction. However, when perfusion drops below the limits of this reserve, that area of brain tissue loses its function and leads to a focal neurological deficit. There is again a range in perfusion where brain tissue could lose function but not necessary undergo necrosis. Thus it is possible for the impaired cerebral function to recover following restoration of perfusion if the area involved has not undergone necrosis and irreversible infarction.
If brain tissue undergoes necrosis and infarction, there is release of chemicals to the surrounding parenchyma resulting in oedema of the white matter that could cause raised ICP and brain displacement. This process could extend the area of brain damage resulting in secondary extension of the infarct. Sometimes, extravasation of blood takes place in the infarcted brain resulting in a haemorrhagic infarct that could further extend the area of brain damage and also further increase ICP. If the infarct and oedema involves the cerebellum, there could be obstruction to CSF pathways resulting in hydrocephalus and raised ICP.

Clinical features
Patients present with a sudden onset of a neurological deficit depending on the area of brain involved. If there is extension of the infarct and brain oedema, they may have raised ICP with impaired consciousness. The location and extent of the infarct is evident on CT scans.

Management
The management of cerebral ischaemia is mainly medical with an attempt to reduce secondary extension of the zone of ischaemia, prevention of further ischaemic episodes and rehabilitation to facilitate recovery from neurological disability.
Surgical interference is indicated in the event of complication such as obstructive hydrocephalus, and heamorrhagic infarction that may sometimes require evacuation to control raised ICP. In case of cerebellar infarction, the swelling of the cerebellum in the restricted confines of the posterior cranial fossa could lead to brain stem compression and respiratory and cardiac dysfunction. In such cases, excision of the infarcted cerebellar tissue helps to control swelling and brain stem compression.
Surgical methods are also employed for revascularisation procedures but more recently endovascular techniques such as angio-plasty are used with increasing frequency.

9

RAISED INTRACRANIAL PRESSURE

Contents

Raised intracranial pressure
   Increase in brain volume
   Increase in CSF volume
   Increase in cerebral blood volume

Raised intracranial pressure,

The normal intracranial pressure (ICP) is 80 - 180mm H_2O or 8 - 13mm Hg. ICP measured via a lumbar puncture (LP) using a spinal manometer is expressed in mm H_2O but this method cannot be used in patients with raised intracranial pressure due to mass lesions because of to the risk of coning. LP manometry may be used only in benign intracranial hypertension where there is no mass lesion or obstructive hydrocephalus causing the raised ICP. In all other instances the ICP is measured via an intracranial transducer introduced via a burr hole. These devices are usually calibrated in mm Hg and the pressure is commonly recorded over a period of time. The pressure thus recorded shows variations synchronous with the arterial pulse and respiratory cycle. The pressure also varies with movement, coughing, breath holding (Valsalva manoeuvre) and pressure on the jugular veins causing venous obstruction (Queckenstedt's test). In patients with raised ICP, abnormal wave forms called Lundberg's A waves are often seen.

The ICP is generated by the contents of the intracranial cavity confined to a closed space within the vault of the skull. The contents are brain (glia 700-900ml, neurons 500-700ml, Extra Cellular Fluid -ECF-100-150ml), blood (100-150ml) and cerebrospinal fluid (CSF 100-150ml) all of which are like water and incompressible but may be displaced. Blood and CSF may be displaced in and out of the intracranial cavity and the brain can displace within the cavity from one compartment to another. In children where the skull bones are not fused, any changes in the volume of the contents would result in an increase in the head size recognized as increasing head circumference. In adults the skull bones are fused and the intracranial contents are enclosed by the rigid vault. Thus, any condition that causes an increase in volume of any of the intracranial contents could result in increased ICP.

The common causes of raised ICP are:

1. Increase of brain volume due to
     cerebral oedema
     space occupying lesions such as tumours, haematomata or abscesses.

2. Increase in CSF volume due to
>   obstruction to the CSF circulation or
>   reduced CSF absorption resulting in hydrocephalus
3. Increase in blood volume due to
>   raised arterial PCO$_2$
>   venous obstruction

1. Increase in brain volume

The normal volume of the brain is 1300 to 1750ml (made up of glia 700-900ml, neurons 500-700ml, Extra Cellular Fluid - ECF 100-150ml). This volume could increase due to a space occupying lesion (SOL) such as a tumour, haematoma or brain abscess or due to cerebral oedema.

There are two types of cerebral oedema, vasogenic and cytotoxic. Vasogenic oedema is seen when fluid accumulates in the interstitial space outside the brain and glial cells (ECF). This form of cerebral oedema is seen in the reaction of the brain to tumours, abscesses, haematomas as well as in over hydration. Cytotoxic oedema where fluid accumulates within the cells is seen when cells are damaged as in cerebral ischaemia or in viral encephalitis.

Raised ICP caused by a space occupying lesion is treated by removing the SOL. Raised ICP due to cerebral oedema is treated with diuretics such as manitol. However, the response of cytotoxic oedema to diurectics is not as good.

2. Increase in CSF volume

The total amount of CSF in the body is about 150 ml, 75 of which is intracranial and 75ml in the spinal subarachnoid space. CSF is produced by the choroid plexus that lies within the ventricular system. CSF flows from the lateral ventricles into the third ventricle through the foramina of Monro and then to the fourth ventricle through the aqueduct of Sylvius. CSF leaves the fourth ventricle via the large midline foramen of Magendie into the cisterna magna and through the small laterally placed foramina of Luschka into the two cerebello-pontine angle cisterns. From the cisterna magna CSF flows down the spinal canal behind the spinal cord and usually ascends in front of the cord to re-enter the intracranial cavity. CSF from the cisterns in the posterior cranial fossa ascends around the brain stem and via the tentorial hiatus to enter the anterior cranial fossa. From here, CSF now ascends over the cerebral hemispheres towards the sagital venous sinus to be absorbed into the blood stream by the arachnoid granulations that protrude into the lateral lacunae of the sinuses.

CSF accumulates either due to obstruction to its circulation or due to reduced absorption. Accumulation of CSF resulting in ventricular dilatation is called hydrocephalus. Increase of CSF production per se does not produce hydrocephalus as the absorbing capacity of the arachnoid granulations far exceeds the capacity to produce. If hydrocephalus results due to an obstruction to CSF circulation before it leaves the fourth ventricle, it is called obstructive hydrocephalus. If hydrocephalus results due to any reason after it has left the fourth ventricle so that the fourth ventricle is in communication with the cisterna magna, it is called a communicating hydrocephalus.
Obstruction to the CSF pathway could occur at any point in its circulation.

The common causes of obstruction are:

Foramen of Monroee
Tumours in the supra-sellar region such as craniopharyngioma, pituitary adenoma and optic nerve glioma that elevate the floor of the third ventricle towards the foramen of Monroe and obstruct the foramen.
Hypothalamic tumours that grow towards the lateral ventricles and occlude the foramina of Monroe.

Third Ventricle
Colloid cyst of third ventricle

Thalamic tumours

Pineal region tumours

Aqueduct of Sylvius
Aqueduct stenosis
Brain stem tumours that distort the aqueduct

Fourth Ventricle
Intra ventricular tumours such as medulloblastoma and ependymoma
Cerebellar tumours, abscesses, haematomas

Cerebellopontine angle tumours
Pontine tumours

Tentorial hiatus
Adhesions due to basal meningitis, commonly tuberculous or fungal

Reduced absorption of CSF occurs due to defects in the arachnoid granulations. These defects could be congenital leading to congenital hydrocephalus where the infant's head enlarges as the ventricles dilate or acquired due to damage to the arachnoid granulations by infections as in neonatal meningitis leading to post meningitic hydrocephalus or due to blood pigment as in spontaneous or traumatic subarachnoid haemorrhage.

Hydrocephalus is treated either by removing an obstruction or bypassing the block. The latter could be achieved by:

a. Ventriculostomy, where a drain is inserted into the ventricle and connected to a closed system.
b. Ventriculo-cisternostomy (Torkildson's operation) where a catheter is inserted in the ventricle and drained into the cisterna magna to bypass a block at the aqueduct.
c. Ventriculoatrial or jugular shunts where a shunt system drains the ventricle to the right atrium or jugular vein.
d. Ventriculoperitoneal shunt which is more commonly used now draining the ventricles to the peritoneal cavity.

3. Increase in cerebral blood volume

The normal cerebral blood volume (CBV) is about 150ml at any given moment. This blood is distributed in the arteries, arterioles, capillaries, venules, veins and the dural sinuses. The arteries are mainly in the base of the brain and branch to supply the brain parenchyma. The veins are thin walled and without valves and could distend easily. As such they act as a reservoir for blood where most of the changes in cerebral blood volume take place. The dural sinuses have rigid walls that do not change much in diameter so that the volume of blood within the sinuses is more or less constant.

As the intracranial cavity is a closed cavity into which blood enters via the arterial system and leaves via the veins, in order to maintain a constant blood volume, the arterial input must exactly balance the venous output. Any discrepancy could cause rapid alterations of blood volume. This balance is maintained by means of the cerebral auto regulation which attempts to maintain a constant blood volume despite wide variations in systemic blood pressure. This mechanism is also independent of the peripheral sympathetic tone and circulating hormones that govern blood flow in other organs. However, cerebral auto regulation is dependent on the partial pressure of arterial CO_2 ($PaCO_2$). Any condition that causes an increase in $PaCO_2$ will result in an increased CBV and if the $PaCO_2$ is reduced, the CBV also decreases.

Increased $PaCO_2$ occurs in surgical patients most commonly due to airway obstruction following aspiration of vomitus, blood, foreign material or if the tongue falls back in an unconscious patient who is improperly positioned supine. Increased $PaCO_2$ could also occur due to concomitant chest complications such as haemothorax, pneumothorax, lung contusions etc. In addition to surgical conditions, $PaCO_2$ could also increase in cyanotic heart disease where venous blood enters the arterial circulation through a reversed cardiac shunt. Arterial $PaCO_2$ can also increase in long standing lung disorders such as emphysema and also in polycythemia where there is an excess of un-oxygenated red cells in circulation. These conditions also cause an increase in CBV leading to raised ICP that result in medical causes of papilloedema.

Raised ICP due to increased blood volume is treated by reducing the $PaCO_2$. This is achieved by correcting airway obstruction as well as by mechanical hyperventilation after paralysing the patient
.

10

CRANIOSPINAL INJURY

Contents

Head Injuries
   Pathophysiology of head injuries
   Secondary brain damage
   Management of patients with head injuries

Spinal injury
   Anatomical considerations
   Mechanism of spinal injury
   Neural injury
   Clinical evaluation
   Management of patients with spinal injuries

Head Injuries

Head injuries constitute a common emergency. In the United Kingdom there are nearly 1 million patients with head injuries seen in the accident and emergency departments each year. Almost half of these are children and males predominate in the ratio two to one. Most head injuries are due to falls (41%) followed by assaults (20%) and road traffic accidents (RTA) (13%). Although RTA account for only 13% of all head injuries attending A&E, they account for 1/3rd of patients transferred for neurosurgical management and also account for 58% of deaths from head injuries. The death rate from head injuries is nine per 100,000 population per year and accounts for 1% of all deaths but 15-20% of deaths in the age range of 5 to 35 years.

Pathophysiology of head injuries
A knowledge of the pathophysiology is essential to understand the management and the outcome of patients with head injuries. There are three basic factors which contribute to the pathophysiology, the forces involved in the process of head injury, the structures damaged and the functional impairment.

Forces
The brain can be injured either when the moving head strikes a stationary object or if a moving object strikes a stationary head. The former is seen in road traffic accidents and in falls and result in deceleration of the head during the impact and the latter in assaults and objects falling on the head leading to acceleration with the impact.

A moving object can strike the stationary head either when the head is supported as could happen when the subject is sleeping or assaulted while pinning the head against the ground. This results in local injuries to the head and the brain called coup injuries and as the head is supported, there may be no acceleration or deceleration of the head and no movement of intra-cranial structures. The object involved could be a sharp object which will penetrate the tissues or a blunt object that tends to crush the tissues. Thus, stab injuries of the head with a sharp weapon could appear quite grotesque but unless a major vessel or vital area of the brain is damaged, neurological function could be well preserved with a good outcome.

A moving object striking the head which is free to move will result in the acceleration of the head, particularly if the object is blunt, rather like a bat striking a ball which then accelerates. During the course of acceleration, due to the different densities of the various intracranial structures, such as bone, white matter, grey matter, cerebrospinal fluid etc, these move at different rates. This results in different relative acceleration forces among these structures rather like shaking a raw egg which leads to disruption of the yolk within with no external evidence of damage to the egg. As a consequence, in addition to the direct injuries sustained at the point of impact, there are injuries to the brain opposite the point of impact resulting in contre-coup injuries, injuries to the brain stem when the hemispheres tend to move on the brain stem held fixed at the tentorial hiatus and also cervical spine injuries when the head moves on the cervical spine. Thus, a single blow could result in multiple intracranial injuries and disruption of neuronal pathways due to internal shear forces resulting in a poor outcome.

When a moving head strikes a stationary object, a similar course of events takes place but in a reverse order due to deceleration of the intracranial structures. The resulting injuries are similar to those produced by acceleration with a similar poor outcome.

A special type of head injury is due to missiles and fire arms. The type of structural damage depends on the velocity of the missile. With low velocity missiles as seen in flying shrapnel during a bomb explosion, there is usually an entrance wound and a track caused by the passage of the missile which is commonly lodged inside. The damage to the brain tends to be restricted to the track and is hence localised. With high velocity missiles as seen in bullets, commonly there is an entrance wound and an exit wound. The dissipation of the energy from the bullet as it passes through the brain causes extensive disruption of nerve tissue similar to an internal explosion resulting in extensive damage to the brain which is often fatal.

The clinical assessment of the forces is possible with an accurate history of the head injury obtained from an eye witness.

Structures damaged
The structures damaged in the course of a head injury may include scalp, skull, meninges and blood vessels, brain, cranial nerves and the cervical spine.

Scalp injuries

Injuries to the scalp can be either open or closed.

Open injuries are scalp lacerations and incised wounds. Unlike skin injuries elsewhere in the body, scalp injuries bleed profusely because the scalp is highly vascular. The blood vessels in the scalp are embedded in the subcutaneous tissue superficial to the galea aponeurotica. The fibrous septa that traverse the subcutaneous tissue attach the skin to the galea preventing incurling of the skin as happens in skin elsewhere and facilitates closure of divided blood vessels. Also, the fibrous septa attach directly to the blood vessels so that after being divided, they are prevented from closing off with spasm and kept open, thus contributing to continuous bleeding from the wound. Such bleeding could be temporarily arrested by pressure on either side of the wound but is best treated with immediate suturing to secure haemostasis until definitive wound toilet is carried out subsequently.

Closed injuries of the scalp are contusions and scalp haematomas where blood collects in the different layers of the scalp. These haematomas can be subcutaneous, sub galeal or subpericranial.
Subcutaneous haematomas appear as painful localised bumps in the scalp as the extravasated blood is localised by the fibrous septa in the subcutaneous tissue.
Subgaleal haematomas spread widely in the vast subgaleal space that extends from the region of the eyebrows up to the occipital region posteriorly, lifting the scalp off the pericranium. The head appears swollen and the scalp fluctuates due to the underlying collection of blood. In small children where the head size is comparatively large in relation to the rest of the body, the volume of blood loss into the subgaleal space can be sufficient to lead to hypovolaemic shock.
Subpericranial haematomas are limited in extent by the attachment of the pericranium along the sutures and hence take the shape of the underlying bone.
Scalp haematomas usually resolve spontaneously but rarely may require aspiration and application of a tight head bandage to prevent recollection.

Skull

Fractures of the skull are simple or compound. Compound fractures can result following damage to the overlying scalp where the fracture is compound to the outside. Skull fractures can also communicate with the exterior at the base of the skull through the para nasal sinuses, pharynx, middle ear and mastoid sinuses and hence be compound from the inside.
Skull fractures are also classified depending on their shape as linear fractures, depressed fractures and comminuted fracture.

Linear fractures per se do not require any special treatment. However, the fact that a patient has sustained such a fracture means that a considerable amount of force has been used and such patients are at risk of developing complications. This risk is increased if the fracture line crosses a vascular marking seen in plain X-ray with the possibility of damage to the underlying blood vessels. Also, the association of a skull fracture with impaired consciousness carries a 25% chance of an intracranial haematoma and such patients require a CT scan to exclude a haematoma.

Depressed fractures carry the risk of damage to the underlying brain. If they are compound, there is an additional risk of foreign material being carried inside with the fractured fragments thus increasing the risk of infection. As such, depressed fractures require surgical excision of the fractured fragments combined with wound toilet if the fracture is compound.

Comminuted fractures where the skull is shattered to several pieces follow head injuries where considerable force has been spent on the skull and usually accompany severe intracranial damage as well.

Meninges and Blood vessels

Damage to the meninges and blood vessels result in the formation of intracranial haematomas. These haematomas can be extradural, subdural or intracerebral. Such haematomas act as space occupying lesions and if sufficiently large, cause raised intra-cranial pressure, brain displacement and herniation and if left untreated, result in death. If the haematoma is small and there is no impairment of consciousness, it can be left to resolve spontaneously.

Heamorrhage into the subarachnoid space following trauma is common leading to traumatic subarachnoid haemorrhage as the blood mixed with CSF does not clot easily. Traumatic SAH does not require special treatment as the blood is soon absorbed but there is a risk of developing communicating hydrocephalus as a late complication.

Damage to the meninges at the base of the skull if accompanied with a fracture would lead to leak of CSF either through the nose causing CSF rhinorrhoea, through the ear causing CSF otorrhoea or into the pharynx. Most CSF leaks heal spontaneously with time but sometimes they require surgical repair if spontaneous closure does not take place.

Brain injury

Injury to the brain can be primary resulting from the forces applied during the course of the injury or secondary due to subsequent complications.

Primary injury could be a contusion or laceration or diffuse axonal injury. Contusion and lacerations can occur directly at the point of impact, opposite the point of impact called contre-coup injuries and at the brain stem due to movement of the hemispheres on the brain stem. Diffuse axonal injury results from shearing forces between grey and white matter which move at different rates during acceleration and deceleration disrupting neuronal pathways.

In contusional injuries, there can be spontaneous resolution of the contusion so that whatever functional disturbances that resulted could potentially recover. Cerebral contusion leads to swelling and discolouration of the brain and the function of the region involved can be disturbed leading to focal neurological deficits.

In cerebral laceration, the functional deficits that ensue are permanent as there is no regeneration of neurons and the effects will depend on the area damaged. Cerebral laceration frequently leads to haemorrhage from the surface of the brain which forms an acute subdural haematoma.

Secondary damage to the brain results due to brain displacement and herniation where there may be haemorrhage around the area involved as seen in the brain stem which becomes distorted with bleeding in the centre.

Herniating brain could also constrict and occlude major arteries leading to infarction as seen in the occipital region with occlusion of the posterior cerebral arteries from transtentorial herniation of the temporal lobes.

Cranial nerves

Cranial nerves can be damaged in the course of a head injury. The commonest to suffer are the olfactory nerves which are slender with a short course through the cribriform plate and antero-posterior movement of the hemispheres with frontal or occipital impacts tend to tear these nerves off resulting in anosmia. The other common nerves to be injured are 7th and 8th nerves due to their long course through a bony canal in the base of the skull and fractures through the skull base could injure these resulting in lower motor neuron facial paralysis, deafness, loss of balance and vertigo. The recovery from nerve injury depends on whether it is neuropraxia, axonotomesis or a neurotomesis..

Cervical spine
The cervical spine is vulnerable to injury when forces are applied to the unsupported head leading to acceleration or deceleration of the head resulting in whiplash injuries. Thus, instability of the cervical spine has to be constantly born in mind when managing patients with head injuries.

Structural damage following a head injury is evaluated by physical examination and investigations such as plain X-rays and CT scans.

Functional disturbance
Injury to the head effects the functioning of the central nervous system depending on the force applied and the structures damaged. One form of functional impairment relates to the structure damaged leading to a corresponding focal neurological deficit. Another form is in relation to the level of consciousness.
If there is no loss of consciousness following a head injury, it can be assumed that the magnitude of the injury is not great and threat to life is minimal. Such patients do not require neurosurgical management and are usually managed with attention to any structural injuries if present.
Sometimes there is a transient loss of consciousness lasting less than about an hour called concussion and here too, the primary damage to the brain is minimal. Such patients require observation at least for 24 hours to be certain that there are no complications. Repeated concussion as in boxers, can have a cumulative effect leading to chronic neuronal loss with time.
If the primary damage is so severe as to involve vital areas of the brain, the injury is usually fatal and such patients commonly succumb at the site. Those who are brought to hospital and ventilated and subsequently found to be brain dead can be candidates for organ donation.
Sometimes, the initial injury causes no loss of consciousness or causes only concussion and the patient initially recovers completely or partially, but after a lucid interval again becomes unconscious. The fact that they first showed signs of recovery means that the primary injury is not severe and has the potential for recovery. The subsequent deterioration is due to secondary factors or complications which are usually preventable or treatable. It is very important that the already damaged brain is protected from additional insult by prevention, early recognition and appropriate management of such complications.

The common complications that can cause secondary brain damage are:

1. Anoxia and hypercapnia will increase the arterial $PaCO_2$ and lead to increased cerebral blood volume and raised intra-cranial pressure that could potentially prove fatal. Thus it is very important to ensure the patency of the upper air way and also to recognise other causes of impaired respiratory function such as associated chest injuries and hypovolaemia and to treat these as a matter of urgency. Regular monitoring of blood gases is essential for patients at risk of developing respiratory complications.

2. Secondary brain damage can also result from raised ICP due to a space occupying lesion such as an intracranial haematoma or hydrocephalus and these can be detected by CT scanning. Those haematomas that are sufficiently large as to cause brain displacement require surgical removal. Sometimes even a relatively small haematoma may cause raised ICP if there is accompanying cerebral oedema and may require removal.

3 Raised ICP can also be caused by cerebral oedema which is evident in the CT scan either

as focal oedema surrounding areas of contusion or more generalised oedema due to diffuse axonal injury. Such patients are usually treated with diuretics such as mannitol, ventilation to control $PaCO_2$ and preferably with continuous monitoring of the ICP with a pressure monitor.

4 Subsequent deterioration of the patient can also occur due to fluid and electrolyte disturbances such as dehydration or over hydration. Patients with head injuries are prone to inappropriate secretion of antidiuretic hormone with a tendency to retain water leading to hyponatraemia. Such complication are detected by frequent monitoring of the fluid balance and electrolytes.

5 Patients with head injuries also deteriorate due to infection. The infection can be intracranial due to post head injury meningitis or a brain abscess or extracranial due to chest infections, urinary infection or gastrointestinal complications resulting in diarrhoea. Usually pyrexia will accompany such an infection. The management consists of prevention of extracranial infections with proper nursing and the early detection and appropriate micro biological evaluation followed by relevant antibiotic therapy in suspected cases.

Functional disturbances are assessed by observation. The parameters observed are:

1. Vital signs (pulse rate, blood pressure, respiratory rate and temperature).
2. Pupillary size and reaction
3 Level of consciousness using the Glasgow coma scale.
4 Neurological deficits
5 Fluid balance and electrolytes

Patients who are unconscious and managed in a neurosurgical intensive care commonly have intracranial pressure monitoring as well as regular blood gas analysis in addition to the observations indicated above. Each time a change suggestive of a deterioration is detected, the patient has to be re-investigated regarding the factors that may be responsible as listed above.

Management of patients with head injuries

It should be born in mind that frequently patients with head injuries may have multiple injuries and some of these may require more urgent attention.

Management of head injured patients consist of:
1. Resuscitation
2. Evaluation
3. Specific surgical procedures
4. Observation
5. Nursing care
6. Rehabilitation

Resuscitation
The first step in the management is to deal with any life threatening conditions using the ATLS principles. Once these are stabilised, the patient has to be assessed regarding the extent of injury, especially stability of the cervical spine and chest, abdominal and limb injuries. Visceral injuries which result in internal haemorrhage require urgent resuscitation and treat-

ment to arrest bleeding. Also chest injuries which impair ventilation lead to a rise in arterial PCO_2 that will cause a catastrophic increase of ICP. Thus, these injuries also have to be attended to first and may require endotracheal intubation and/or chest drains to ensure adequate ventilation.

Evaluation
After initial resuscitation, the patient should be evaluated regarding the forces that caused the injury, the structural damage and the functional disturbances. This is done with a detailed history of the injury obtained from an eye witness and others concerned with the initial management and transport such as ambulance crew or paramedics. A complete neurological examination followed by plain X-rays and CT scans where indicated will outline the extent of structural damage.

Specific Surgical procedures
Surgical treatment is planned depending on the extent of injuries and involves management of scalp wounds, skull fractures or any intracranial haematomas. Open scalp wounds require proper wound toilet, haemostasis and repair. Compound depressed fractures also require wound toilet and often excision of the fractured bone fragments and repair of any dural tears. In uncontaminated depressed fractures, the bone fragments can be replaced. Bone defects left due to excision of bone fragments are later repaired with a prosthesis. An intracranial haematoma may require evacuation if it significantly raises ICP. If CSF continues to leak from the nose or rarely the ear, this requires surgical repair to prevent meningitis.

Observation
The patient is then observed regarding further progress. Neurological observations are carried out as frequently as deemed necessary. In the event of any deterioration, the patient has to be re-investigated to exclude any complications as mentioned above and if such a complication is detected, appropriately treated.

Nursing care
Proper nursing care is of paramount importance to ensure recovery of the damaged neural structures with attention to fluid balance, nutrition and physiotherapy. In unconscious patients, particular attention has to be directed towards prevention of complications such as hypostatic and aspiration pneumonia, urinary and gastro-intestinal infections and skin care. In the event of major neurological deficits, planned rehabilitation is essential to ensure useful recovery of function.

Rehabilitation
Many patients with structural damage to the brain are left with disabling neurological deficits and require rehabilitation to facilitate further improvement. The neurological disability could be assessed and subsequently monitored using a numerical disability scale.

Spinal injury

Spinal injury is important due to the potential threat to life as well as the risk of serious disability.

Anatomical considerations

The vertebral column forms a strut which provides support to the body structures and also affords protection to the spinal cord and cauda equina traversing the spinal canal. The spinal column is made up of several segments in the form of vertebral bodies that are stacked on top of each other forming a continuous bony canal containing the spinal cord and cauda equina. This arrangement provides protection to the neural structures while permitting mobility of the trunk. To ensure this dual function of protection of the neural structures as well as mobility within a certain range, it is necessary for the spinal column to be stable. This stability is ensured by:

1. Bony configuration
2. Joints
3. Ligaments
4. Muscles

Bony configuration
Each vertebra is made up of the vertebral body that forms the main strut and the posterior aspect of the vertebral body, pedicles and lamina form the spinal canal. The bony configuration of the vertebrae permit them to be stacked on top of each other to make the vertebral column and the spinal canal for the passage of the neural structures.

Joints
Each vertebra is linked to the adjacent vertebrae with the intervertebral joint anteriorly between the two vertebral bodies and two pairs of apophyseal joints posteriorly.
The intervertebral joints are made of the intervertebral disc which has a tough annulus fibrosus that forms a ring enclosing the softer nucleus pulposus. This arrangement permits tilting movement similar to a ball bearing while preventing lateral dislocation and also acts as a shock absorber during vertical impact.
The apophyseal joints posteriorly are synovial joints that permit rotation of the spine and their configuration in different parts of the spine imposes a limit to the degree of rotation permitted at that level.

Ligaments
Several ligaments serve to bind one vertebra to another and those important for stability are the anterior longitudinal ligament, the posterior longitudinal ligament, ligamentum flavum and inter-spinous ligaments.

Muscles
The posterior and anterior para-spinal muscles which are concerned with movement of the spine also contribute to the stability especially in the event of injury. The pain resulting from a spinal injury causes reflex contraction of the paraspinal muscles that prevent further movement of the spine. This factor is important when moving patients with spinal injury especially under anaesthesia where stability of the spine maintained with muscle contraction can be

lost during anaesthesia resulting in instability that could damage the spinal cord.

The three column concept
The anatomical structures affecting the stability of the spine could be resolved into three columns and this concept has been useful in the evaluation of patients with spinal injury concerning their stability. The anterior column consists of the anterior longitudinal ligament and the anterior vertebral body complex, the middle column is made of the posterior longitudinal ligament, annulus and posterior vertebral body complex, and the posterior column comprises of the facet joints, ligamentum flavum, laminae, posterior spinous processes and interspinous ligaments.

Mechanism of spinal injury
The part of the spine most likely to be injured are the portions that are most mobile such as the cranio-vertebral junction, cervical spine and the dorso-lumbar spine. The type of spinal injury can be classified depending on the different forces to flexion injuries, extension injuries, vertical compression injuries, flexion rotation injuries and penetrating injuries.

Flexion injuries
Forces that cause excessive flexion of the spine tend to crush the vertebral body deforming it to a wedge shape (anterior wedge compression fracture). Such injuries result during acute flexion of the which can occur when heavy objects fall on the head flexing the neck or during diving into shallow water. Sometimes, acute flexion distracts the posterior elements of the spine (flexion distraction injuries) causing a tear of the interspinous ligaments, fracture of the spinous processes which could extend to the laminae and the pedicles and even damage the annulus posteriorly resulting in traumatic disc protrusion. The stability of the spine is largely maintained in wedge compression fractures but could be compromised if there is extensive damage to the posterior column. This could occur in flexion distraction injuries which sometimes cause subluxation without a fracture more commonly seen in the cervical spine.

Extension injuries
Extension injuries result during whip lash and also falling on the chin. These injuries are common in the cervical spine and the anterior longitudinal ligaments are torn with damage to the anterior aspect of the intervertebral disc that tends to open out in front. The posterior structures are compressed and could result in fracture of the laminae. These fractures are also stable to a large extent but could become unstable in the long term resulting in spondylolisthesis.

Vertical compression injuries.
Vertical compression injuries follow vertical impact on the spine such as falling from a height on to the buttocks. The lumbar spine is more prone to this sort of injury and results in collapse of the vertebral body or a burst fracture. Such injuries are usually stable but could result in damage to the spinal cord from bone fragments or haematoma.

Flexion rotation injuries
Flexion rotation injuries result during major trauma such as road accidents. They cause damage to more than one column and fractures could involve the vertebral bodies as well as the pedicles and result in instability of the spine. Often the spine could be completely dislocated with irreversible damage to the spinal cord.

Penetrating injuries
Penetrating injuries could be due to stab injuries, gun shot or missile wounds. Stab injuries could transect the spinal cord without much injury to the spine or causing instability. The transection could be incomplete resulting in a Brown Sequard syndrome or complete resulting in paraplegia or quadruplegia. Gun shot and missile injuries damage the spinal cord and/or the spine and could result in instability of the spine depending on the extent of damage.

Neural injury

The dreaded complication of a spinal injury is the damage to neural structures such as spinal cord, cauda equina and nerve roots.

The mechanism of injury to neural elements could be :

1. Transection during
   (a) penetrating injuries.
   (b) spinal dislocation.

2. Compression from
   (a) Deformed or narrowed spinal canal
   (b) Fractured bone fragments
   (c) Herniated disc material
   (d) Haematoma

3. Ischaemia
   (a) Injury to the anterior spinal artery
   (b) Injury to important radicular arteries
   (c) Prolonged compression

4. Secondary damage during movement of a patient with an unstable spinal injury where the mobile fragments cause injury to the spinal cord which may have been spared during the initial injury.

5. Central cord haemorrhage resulting in the central cord syndrome commonly following injury to the spinal cord from osteophytes during an extension injury.

Sequelae of neural injury

Injury to the neural elements such as the spinal cord, cauda equina or nerve roots result in impairment of motor, sensory and autonomic function below the level of the lesion.

Motor function
Spinal cord injury could result in weakness or paralysis of all muscle groups below the level of the lesion. If the injury involves the spinal cord, initially there is period of spinal shock during which period there is a flaccid weakness of all the muscles below the level of the lesion. As the stage of spinal activity returns, the muscle tone increases and becomes spastic with increased tendon reflexes and a tendency to spontaneous flexor spasms. With long standing spasticity, contractures of the limb with fixed deformities could develop.
If the injury involves the cauda equina, the weakness is lower motor neuron with reduced muscle tone and progressive muscle wasting.
In the case of cervical injuries, respiratory function could be impaired due to paralysis of

intercostal muscles and if the lesion is above C3 or 4, paralysis of the diaphragm could occur leading to respiratory arrest.

Sensory function
Following injury, superficial as well as deep sensations are impaired below the level of the lesion. This is usually evident as a sensory level during neurological examination. With recovery, there could be altered and abnormal sensations such as allodynia which is a very unpleasant feeling of pain during non noxious stimulation. A late sequelae is paraplegic pain which is again very difficult to treat. Such pain syndromes are due to de-afferentiation of the sensory pathways.

Autonomic function
Disturbed autonomic function could involve the urinary bladder, bowel, sexual function in males, peripheral vascular bed, cardiac function, sweating and piloerection.
Initially there is a period of urinary retention. In injuries involving the spinal cord, with return of reflex activity following the initial period of spinal shock, reflex bladder function becomes evident whereas with a cauda equina injury, the bladder remains non contractile. There is frequently constipation that require proper management of bowel function. In males sexual function could be impaired leading to loss of erection, loss of ejaculation or sometimes priapism.

Involvement of the sympathetic outflow following cervical injuries result in bradycardia and hypotension. Hypotension is due to loss of sympathetic tone in the peripheral vessels and fall in peripheral resistance and impaired cardiac output. With the onset of reflex spinal cord activity there could be altered autonomic states resulting in autonomic dysreflexia where there could be catastrophic episodes of hypertension especially during bladder distention. Impaired sweating could result in hyper-pyrexia especially with high spinal cord lesions.

Pressure sores
In paralysed patients, the combination of loss of sensations and loss of vascular tone and stagnation of the microcirculation make the skin prone to pressure sores.

Clinical evaluation

Evaluation of the patient is directed towards
    a. Identification and prevention of life threatening situations
    b. Assessment of extent of injury and neurological function
    c. Assessment of stability of the spine and integrity of the spinal cord

a. Identification and prevention of life threatening situations
This is mainly first aid with attention to airway, breathing and circulation. With multiple injuries visible bleeding requires to be arrested with direct pressure.
The vital signs are important as damage to the sympathetic outflow in a high cervical spine lesion could cause bradycardia, hypotension and hyperpyrexia from absent sweating. Respiration may be inadequate due to intercostal muscle paralysis and if the lesion is above C4, the diaphragm could also be paralysed resulting in apnoea.
b. Assessment of extent of injury and neurological function
A detailed history will serve to outline the forces involved in the injury which in turn will

indicate the possibility of an unstable injury.
Examination is directed towards general assessment of the patient regarding other injuries, examination of the spine regarding the site of the injury and local deformities and identification of any neurological deficits.

c. Assessment of stability of the spine and integrity of the spinal cord
Radiological examination with plain X-rays often confirms the spinal injury and also serve to assess stability of the spine. Injuries involving more than 1 column are potentially unstable. CT scans of the spine across the region of injury are useful to evaluate the extent of bony damage and also displacement of the fracture fragments. MRI is useful to identify the extent of neural injury especially with regard to the extent of spinal cord damage and also outline any compressive element.

Management of patients with spinal injuries

The aims of management are
1. Prevention of secondary damage to the spinal cord during movement
2. Relief of spinal cord compression if any
3. Stabilisation of the spine
4. Prevention and management of complications of neural injury
5. Rehabilitation

1. Prevention of secondary damage to the spinal cord during movement
Where a spinal injury is suspected, particular attention is required in terms of movement of the patient to avoid secondary damage to the spinal cord from an unstable injury of the spine. This is especially important in moving the neck attempting to maintain the airway and the patient should be turned as a whole without moving the neck only.

2. Relief of spinal cord compression
Spinal cord compression could be caused by protruded disc material, bone fragments, haematoma or by the deformity of the spinal canal. Such compression could cause a neurological deficit which is potentially reversible if there is no damage to the spinal cord itself. Where spinal cord compression is identified, urgent surgical decompression could facilitate recovery of impaired neurological function.

3. Stabilisation of the spine
In the event of instability of the spine, stabilisation is required. This could be achieved either with external means or internally and the method used also depends on the site of injury. The sites of injury could be cranio-vertebral junction, cervical spine and dorso-lumbar spine.

a. Craniovertebral junction
Injuries to the craniovertebral junction in the form of fractures and/or dislocations involve the atlas, axis and the atlanto-occipital joint in different combinations and are often fatal or life threatening. Stabilisation could be achieved externally with the use of a halo-vest or internally with many of the recent metal implants that are now available.

b. Cervical spine injuries
Stable injuries of the cervical spine are often treated with a cervical collar mainly for comfort. Unstable injuries require external stabilisation with a halo-vest or internal fixation with metal devices and bone graft.

c. Injuries to the dorso-lumbar spine
Stable injuries of the dorso-lumbar spine may be treated with a jacket mainly for comfort but unstable injuries require internal fixation with metal devices and bone graft.

4. Prevention and management of complications of neural injury
The complications of neural injury are the result of motor, sensory and autonomic dysfunction below the level of the lesion.

Motor dysfunction leads to paralysis which is initially flaccid. In the case of spinal cord injury, the limbs become spastic with return of reflex activity after initial period of spinal shock but in the case of cauda equina injury, the tone remains flaccid with progressive wasting of the muscles. Poor management in the initial period could result in gross deformities of the limbs due to contractures and ankylosis of joints and the prevention of these require early institution of dedicated physiotherapy. Early rehabilitation serves to improve mobility using devices such as wheel chairs and walking appliances.

Sensory dysfunction together with loss of movement and poor skin circulation due to autonomic disturbances lead to the formation of pressure sores. Dedicated nursing which includes the use of special beds is required to prevent this dreaded complication which sometimes could prove fatal.

Autonomic dysfunction impairs bladder, bowel and sexual function as well as the circulation and attention to these is another component of nursing and medical care. Impaired bladder function may result in recurrent urinary infections, hydronephrosis and renal failure which is a common cause of mortality among paraplegic patients. Proper attention to bladder and bowel function with monitoring of renal function is essential to prevent these complications.

5. Rehabilitation
Rehabilitation constitutes the mainstay of management of those patients with neural injury. The aim of rehabilitation is to return the patient to the society with much functional and psychological independence as possible and requires the concerted efforts of physiotherapists, psychotherapists and occupational therapists and medical personnel to achieve this goal.

11

DISEASES OF THE SPINE

Contents

Spinal cord compression
Degenerative disease of the spine
Cervical spondylosis
Lumbar spondylosis

Spinal cord compression

Spinal cord compression is a common neurosurgical emergency and requires a proper understanding of the pathophysiology and prompt attention if irreversible damage and consequent life long paralysis is to be avoided.

The spinal cord extends from the foramen magnum down to about the lower border of L1 vertebra and lesions causing cord compression have to be situated in this region. Lesions below L1 cause compression of the cauda equina leading to a lower motor neurone paralysis of the lower limbs.

Pathophysiology
Compression of the spinal cord results in impairment of function of the spinal cord below the level of the lesion. The functions thus affected are:

1. Motor function resulting in weakness of the lower limbs, spasticity, increased reflexes and an extensor plantar response.
2. Sensory function resulting in loss of superficial as well as deep sensation below the level of the lesion.
3. Autonomic function resulting in loss of bladder and bowel control and in males lack of erection and ejaculation, loss of vascular tone, loss of sweating and loss of piloerection. Lesions above T1 also cause disturbances of cardiac function and blood pressure due to sympathetic paralysis.

The disturbance of spinal cord function during compression is due to many factors:
1. There is an element of mechanical compression of the white matter tracts that lead to impaired function.

2. In addition there is a vascular element where the venous drainage from the area of compression is impaired leading to venous stasis and oedema of the spinal cord which could later lead to a venous infarct. There could also be arterial compression leading to ischaemia and infarction.

3. Certain lesions such as malignant deposits and infections cause an endarteritis resulting in thrombosis of the blood vessels and spinal cord ischaemia.

4. In other instances, chemicals which are neurotoxic such as vasogenic amines are released by the compressivve lesion especially in malignant deposits with tumour necrosis, which directly damage the spinal cord.

5. Certain lesions cause destruction of the vertebral column that could lead to instability. The abnormal movements which result due to the instability could also inflict mechanical injury to the spinal cord.

The altered function of the spinal cord could be reversed with relief of the compression leading to restoration of function only if the cord had not been irreversibly damaged. If the period, nature and extend of compression are such that the spinal cord has been permanently damaged, surgical relief of compression is unlikely to restore function.

Causes of spinal cord compression

Lesions causing compression of the spinal cord could be extradural, intradural but extramedullary or intramedullary.

Extradural lesions
Extradural lesions arise from the different tissues in the extradural space.

Fat	-Lipomas
Blood vessels	-Angiomas, Dural A-V fistulas
Nerves	-Neurofibroma
Meninges	-Meningioma
Intervertebral discs	- Disc protrusion
Vertebral bodies	-Congenital malformations of the spine
	-Traumatic lesions due to blood clots or bone fragments
	-Acute infections such as epidural abscesses
	-Chronic infections such as tuberculosis
	-Primary bone tumours such as myeloma, osteoclastoma, osteosarcoma, and haemangioma.
	-Metastases from midline organs such as thyroid, oesophagus, stomach, pancreas, cervix and prostate and from paired organs such as bronchi, breast, kidneys, ovaries and testes.

Intradural but extramedullary lesions
The common lesions are meningiomas and neurofibromas.

Intramedullary lesions
The common lesions within the spinal cord are

1. Primary spinal cord tumours such as astrocytomas and ependymomas.
2. Metastasis into the spinal cord from other organs and melanomas.

3. Infections such as abscess, parasitic cysts or tuberculomas.
4. Syringomyelia, either spontaneous or post traumatic
5. Haematomas, spontaneous or traumatic.

Clinical Features.
The clinical features have been described in detail in the chapter on paraplegia in the neurology section. The symptoms are impaired sensation, paraesthesiae and numbness below the level of the lesion, weakness and/or stiffness of the limbs, and loss of bladder, bowel or sexual function. If the lesion is below the cervical spine, the symptoms will be confined to the trunk and lower limbs but if the lesion involves the cervical spine, the symptoms would involve the upper limbs as well.

The onset will depend on the type of lesion and would be sudden in vascular diseases, progressive in tumours, following injury in traumatic lesions, with fever and rapid ill health in infections and apparent at birth in congenital lesions.

Examination may reveal a spinal deformity or local tenderness at the site of the lesion. The neurological deficits would be sensory impairment often with a sensory level corresponding to the site of the lesion and weakness of the limbs below the site of the lesion. If the lesion is acute in onset, often there is hypotonia with diminished reflexes but in long standing lesions, there is spasticity with exaggerated reflexes. If the lesion involves the cauda equina, the weakness of the lower limbs would flaccid be with reduced tone and reflexes and a segmental type of sensory disturbance.

Investigations
First line investigation in suspected spinal cord compression are plain X-rays at the relevant clinical level and ESR and/or CRP. The ESR is raised in cord compression due to lesions destroying the bone and also in infective lesions. Plain X-rays reveal evidence of bone destruction or other bone changes in long standing lesions such as scalloping of the vertebral bodies and also the soap bubble appearance seen in vertebral haemangiomas. Plain X-rays also are helpful in assessing the stability of the spine.

Specialised investigations designed to outline the compressing lesion are CT scans, myelography with or without CT and MRI. MRI is the most helpful in that it enables sagittal views of the spinal cord and also evidence of spinal cord involvement apparent as signal change within the cord.

Management
The aims of management are to relieve the spinal cord compression by surgical decompression, stabilise the spine where necessary, promote neurological recovery and treat any underlying disorder.

Surgical decompression
The technique of surgical decompression depends on the type of compression encountered and the nature of the lesion. Intramedullary and intradural extramedullary compression require a laminectomy or laminoplasty. For extradural compression, the choice of operation depends on the type of lesion involved. If the compression is anterior, the spine may have to approached anteriorly either through the neck or through the thorax or in the case of thoracic compression, postero-laterally by removing the appropriate transverse process and portion of rib (costo-transversectomy). If the lesion has caused destabilisation of the spine, it may have to combined with an internal fixation procedure which usually involves bone grafts and/or implants. Surgical decompression also gives the opportunity for a histological diagnosis that

is important to plan further treatment. Stabilisation of the spine is achieved by external devices such as a halo-vest in the case of the cervical spine or internal devices such as plates and screws or rods.

Treatment of the underlying disorder
This depends on the cause of spinal cord compression. If the compression is due to an infection, this has to be appropriately treated with antibiotics. If it is a malignant lesion, management consists of treating the underlying malignancy with radiotherapy and/or chemotherapy. Sometimes, the nature of the lesion is such that surgical decompression may not be the best option due to extensive disease or the general state of the patient. In such instances, histological diagnosis could, be achieved by radiologically aided percutaneous biopsy of the lesion and appropriate treatment planned depending on the histological findings.

Promotion of neurological recovery.
The ultimate aim is to promote neurological recovery so that the patient will regain lost function and will be restored to normal mobility and normal bowel and bladder function. This requires prevention of complications such as pressure sores and urinary and gastro-intestinal infection with dedicated nursing followed by a period of physiotherapy and rehabilitation to mobilise the patient. If the spinal cord is damaged beyond repair, the patient will need a complete course of rehabilitation in order to manage in a wheel chair with attention to bladder and bowel function as well.

Degenerative disease of the spine

Degenerative disease of the spine affects mainly the cervical and the lumber regions which are the most mobile parts of the spine. Such degenerative changes result in cervical or lumbar spondylosis.

Cervical spondylosis
Cervical spondylosis is the result of degenerative changes which primarily affects the joints in the cervical spine.

Pathophysiology
Each vertebral body has 2 pairs of apophyseal joints and an inter vertebral joint. The apophyseal joints are synovial joints and are placed posteriorly. The paravertebral muscles are attached to the joint capsule which also has a rich nerve supply from the posterior primary rami of the cervical nerves. These joints are incorporated in the boundary of the inter vertebral foramina through which the nerve roots exit and the radicular arteries and veins traverse. They also are incorporated into the boundaries of the spinal canal which contains the spinal cord.

The intervertebral discs are placed anteriorly between two vertebral bodies and consist of a thick fibrous annulus fibrosus which encloses a soft nucleus pulposus. The spinal canal is formed by the posterior aspects of the vertebral bodies and intervertebral discs anteriorly, the pedicles and the apophyseal joints laterally and the laminae posteriorly. The bony structures that form the spinal canal are covered anteriorly by the posterior longitudinal ligament and posteriorly by the ligamentum flavum. The intervertebral foramina which the nerve roots and radicular vessels traverse are formed by the lateral aspect of the inter vertebral discs, the pedicles, a part of the vertebral body and the apophyseal joints. The vertebral artery traverses the foramina transversaria.

Cervical spondylosis which primarily affects the apophyseal joints and the intervertebral joints hence influence the paravertebral muscles, the ligaments of the spine, the spinal canal and hence the spinal cord and the intervertebral foramina and therefore the neurovascular structures that pass through them and also the vertebral artery. Involvement of the apophyseal joints result in arthritic changes that cause swelling of the joints and pain. This pain also results in contraction of the paravertebral muscles leading to a stiff neck. The joint swelling could influence the nerve root that exit the relevant intervertebral foramen causing the pain to radiate down the arm often with paraesthesiae in the distribution of the nerve root. With chronic apophyseal joint disease, there is thickening of the articular surfaces and hence the joint itself. The thickened joint encroaches into the intervertebral foramen leading to mechanical nerve root compression leading to sensory and motor disturbances of the area supplied by that nerve root. Stenosis of the intervertebral foramen also influences the venous drainage and the arterial supply of the spinal cord via the radicular vessels and contribute to the myelopathy that affects the spinal cord.

The hypertrophied joints also encroach on the spinal canal resulting in stenosis of the spinal canal and mechanical compression of the spinal cord leading to spinal cord dysfunction. Involvement of the intervertebral joints causes weakness of the annulus fibrosus which tends to bulge outwards. Bulging of the annulus towards the intervertebral foramen results in narrowing of the foramen and nerve root compression and bulging towards the spinal canal contributes to the spinal stenosis. Abnormal vascularisation could occur in relation to the degenerated intervertebral discs resulting in the formation of osteophytes that also contribute to narrowing of the spinal canal and intervertebral foramina. The degenerate annulus can rupture leading to extrusion of the nucleus pulposus. If the nucleus is extruded towards the intervertebral foramen, the nerve root would be compressed resulting in acute brachalgia and nerve root dysfunction. If the nucleus is extruded towards the spinal canal, acute spinal cord compression could occur.

With degenerative changes in the intervertebral joints, there is reduction of the height of the discs and if several discs are involved, the height of the entire cervical spine would be significantly reduced. As the spine becomes shorter, the ligamentum flavum tends to buckle and encroach on the diameter of the spinal canal leading to spinal stenosis. Degenerative changes could also affect the anterior and posterior longitudinal ligaments which become weak leading to instability of the cervical spine. There is a tendency for subluxation of the vertebral bodies and this too contributes to the spinal canal stenosis. Instability of the cervical spine could also compromise the blood flow in the vertebral arteries leading to vertebro-basilar ischaemia.

Thus, with cervical spondylosis, there is a radiculopathy due to stenosis of the intervertebral foramina which is a result of hypertrophy of the apophyseal joints, bulging of the annulus fibrosus and osteophyte formation. Acute disc protrusion into the intervertebral foramen could result in acute nerve root compression. Cervical spondylosis could also result in a myelopathy which follows compression of the spinal cord by stenosis of the spinal canal due to the hypertrophied apophyseal joints, bulging annulus, osteophytes and buckling of the ligamentum flavum. Myelopathy is also caused by instability of the cervical spine due to degenerate ligaments. Narrowing of the intervertebral foramina can lead to vascular disturbances in the spinal cord and result in venous engorgement or arterial insufficiency which also contributes to the myelopathy. Acute disc protrusion into the spinal canal could lead to acute cord compression. There may be vertebro-basilar ischaemia due to instability of the cervical spine.

Clinical features

The clinical features depend on the extent of the disease and involvement of the nerve roots leading to a radiculopathy and the spinal cord leading to a myelopathy. Neck pain and stiffness are commonly the first symptoms when the apophyseal joints are swollen and the para vertebral muscles are contracted. The pain often radiates to the upper limb and may be accompanied by paraesthesiae. There may be local tenderness over the apophyseal joints with restriction of cervical spine movements. With advanced radiculopathy, lower motor neurone signs appear in the upper limbs in a segmental distribution with weakness and wasting of muscles. There can be a corresponding sensory deficit in the distribution of the relevant nerve root. With acute disc protrusion, acute brachialgia follows with severe pain radiating down the upper limb with sensory and motor changes in a segmental distribution.

Myelopathy results in an upper motor neurone type of weakness in the lower limbs with spasticity, weakness and brisk tendon reflexes. There may be bladder and bowel disturbances but this is uncommon. Sensory changes may be elicited in the trunk and lower limbs. With instability of the cervical spine, flexion of the neck can result in a Lhermitte's sign with electric shock like sensations felt down the body. Sometimes, instability may compromise blood flow in the vertebral arteries resulting in vertebro-basilar ischaemia and episodes of dizziness with neck movements.

Investigations

Plain X-rays are useful to reveal the degenerative changes in the spine. Flexion and extension views help to establish instability indicated by subluxation of the vertebral bodies during flexion. Narrowing of the intervertebral foramina or the spinal canal or the presence of disc protrusion is best revealed by CT scans, MRI scans or CT myelogram. MRI scans are useful to demonstrate the extent of myelopathy which is evident as signal change within the spinal cord.

Management

Management depends on the clinical presentation. Symptoms such as pain due to apophyseal joint disease are managed with analgesics and muscle relaxants such as diasepam. Radicular pain responds to amitryptiline or anticonvulsants such as carbamazepine. Adjuvant methods such as physiotherapy are often useful. Surgical treatment is indicated in case of nerve root or spinal cord compression and in cervical instability. Acute disc protrusion requires urgent surgical decompression of the spinal cord and/or nerve roots. Chronic compression of the nerve roots is treated with foraminotomy where the narrowed intervertebral foramen is enlarged by removing the bony roof. Chronic spinal cord compression and myelopathy are treated with anterior decompression of the involved segment by removing the intervertebral disc anteriorly via an incision in the neck. The decompressed segment can be fused with a bone graft or left as it is. If there is instability, the involved vertebral bodies are further stabilised with implants using plates and screws. If there is extensive stenosis of the spinal canal, especially with buckling of the ligamentum flavum, cervical laminectomy may be indicated.

Lumbar spondylosis

Degenerative changes involving the lumbo-sacral spine lead to lumbar spondylosis.

Pathophysiology
The pathophysiological changes affecting the lumbar spine are similar to that in the cervical spine. However, the anatomy is different in that there is no spinal cord in the lumbar region and narrowing of the spinal canal leads to compression of the cauda equina.
Lumbar spondylosis affects the apophyseal joints and the intervertebral joints and influences the paravertebral muscles, the ligaments of the spine, the spinal canal and hence the cauda equina and the intervertebral foramina and the nerve roots that pass through them.

Involvement of the apophyseal joints result in arthritic changes that cause swelling of the joints and pain. This pain results in contraction of the paravertebral muscles leading to a stiff back. The joint swelling could influence the nerve root that exit the relevant intervertebral foramen causing the pain to radiate down the lower limb commonly called sciatica, as well as producing paraesthesiae in the distribution of the nerve root. With chronic apophyseal joint disease, there is thickening of the articular surfaces and hence the joint itself. The thickened joint encroaches into the intervertebral foramen leading to mechanical nerve root compression leading to sensory and motor disturbances of the segment supplied by that nerve root. The hypertrophied joints also encroaches into the spinal canal resulting in stenosis of the spinal canal and compression of the cauda equina. Involvement of the intervertebral joints cause weakness of the annulus fibrosus which tends to bulge outwards. Bulging of the annulus towards the intervertebral foramen results in narrowing of the foramen and nerve root compression and bulging towards the spinal canal contributes to the spinal stenosis. Abnormal vascularisation could occur in relation to the degenerated intervertebral discs resulting in the formation of osteophytes that also contribute to narrowing of the spinal canal and intervertebral foramina.

The degenerate annulus can rupture leading to extrusion of the nucleus pulposus. If the nucleus is extruded towards the intervertebral foramina, the nerve roots would be compressed resulting in acute sciatica and nerve root dysfunction. If the nucleus is extruded towards the spinal canal, acute cauda equina compression could occur. With degenerative changes in the intervertebral joints, there is reduction of the height of the discs and also hypertrophy of the ligamentum flavum. This also encroaches into the diameter of the spinal canal leading to spinal stenosis. Degenerative changes could also affect the anterior and posterior longitudinal ligaments which become weak leading to instability of the lumbar spine, a tendency for subluxation and spondylolisthesis.

Thus, with lumbar spondylosis, there is a radiculopathy due to stenosis of the intervertebral foramina which is a result of hypertrophy of the apophyseal joints, bulging of the annulus fibrosus and osteophyte formation. Acute lateral disc protrusion towards the intervertebral foramina could result in acute nerve root compression and sciatica. Lumbar spondylosis could also result in stenosis of the spinal canal due to the hypertrophied apophyseal joints, bulging annulus, osteophytes and thickened ligamentum flavum. This impairs the functioning of the cauda equina and leads to intermittent claudication. Acute central disc protrusion into the spinal canal could result in acute cauda equina compression resulting in a cauda equina syndrome. Cauda equina compression could also occur with advanced spondylolisthesis.

Clinical features

The clinical features depend on the extent of the disease and involvement of the nerve roots and of the cauda equina. Low back pain and sciatica are commonly the first symptoms when the apophyseal joints are swollen and the para vertebral muscles are contracted. The pain may be accompanied by paraesthesiae and there may be local tenderness over the apophyseal joints with restriction of lumbar spine movements. With nerve root compression there is segmental weakness and sensory impairment in the distribution of the relevant nerve root. Stretching the nerve root by elevating the limb causes pain recognised as limitation in the straight leg raising test.

Spinal canal stenosis presents with intermittent claudication which is very similar to ischaemic claudication but without any evidence of limb ischaemia. It is hence called neurogenic intermittent claudication and may or may not be accompanied by neurological deficits. Cauda equina compression occurs with acute central disc protrusion and leads to distal weakness in the lower limbs with flaccidity and absent tendon reflexes. There is commonly bladder and bowel disturbances with lax sphincters and sensory changes involving the saddle area. With instability of the lumbar spine and spondylolisthesis, chronic cauda equina compression could occur with progressive lower limb weakness and impaired bladder and bowel function.

Investigations

Plain X-rays are useful to reveal the degenerative changes in the spine. Flexion and extension views help to establish instability indicated by subluxation of the vertebral bodies during flexion. Narrowing of the intervertebral foramina or the spinal canal or the presence of disc protrusion is best revealed by CT scans, MRI scans or CT myelogram.

Management

Management depends on the clinical presentation. Symptoms such as pain due to apophyseal joint disease are managed with analgesics and muscle relaxants such as diazepam. Radicular pain responds to amitryptiline or anticonvulsants such as carbamazepine. Adjuvant methods such as local heat, correction of posture and physiotherapy are often useful.

Surgical treatment is indicated in case of nerve root or cauda equina compression and in lumbar instability and spondylolisthesis. Acute disc protrusion requires urgent surgical decompression of the cauda equina and/or nerve roots. Chronic lateral disc protrusion causing compression of the nerve roots is treated with excision of the disc (microdiscectomy). Narrow foramina may require enlargement of the lateral recess by removing the bony roof. Chronic spinal stenosis is treated with laminectomy or laminotomy. If there is instability, the involved vertebral bodies are further stabilised with interbody bone grafts or pedicle crews.

12

NERVE ENTRAPMENT AND DISORDERS OF PERIPHERAL NERVES

Contents

Introduction
Nerve injuries
Entrapment neuropathies
Peripheral nerve compression

Introduction
Peripheral nerves are bundles of axons encased in a myelin sheath. Thus they are long prolongations of a centrally placed cell body and disorders of the peripheral nerves affect the entire unit which includes the cell body, the axon tube and the target of innervation. The axons in the peripheral nerve are covered with a sheath called the endoneurium and arranged in bundles to form fascicles. Each fascicle is covered with a perineurium and the fascicles are in turn arranged in several bundles enclosed in another sheath called the epineureum which is the outermost covering of a peripheral nerve. The peripheral nerves are often mixed containing motor, sensory and autonomic nerves and also incorporates blood vessels that supply the nerve called a vasa nervorum, lymphatics and also sensory nerves endings called the nervi nervorum.

Peripheral nerve disorders encountered in neurosurgical practice are

1. Nerve injuries
2. Entrapment neuropathies
3. Nerve compression by tumours

Nerve injuries

Mechanism
Peripheral nerves can be injured in different forms

a. Laceration of nerves occur with cut injuries involving soft tissues.
b. Focal contusion is commonly seen in gun shot and missile injuries
c Stretch or traction injuries occur when a nerve is stretched as in the brachial plexus.

d. Compression of a nerve is seen in Saturday night palsy and due to an ill-fitting plaster cast.
e. Drug injection injury when drugs are inadvertently injected into nerves
f. Electrical injury during contact with high tension wires.

Pathophysiology
Following injury to the peripheral nerve, changes occur in the cell body proximally, in the axon tube and in the muscle innervated distally.

In the cell body there is chromatolysis with displacement of the Nissl substance to the periphery of the cell.

In the axon, Wallerian degeneration occurs up to the first Node of Ranvier proximally and along the entire length of the nerve distally. The axon and myelin degenerate and are removed by phagocytes leaving empty endoneureal tubes. The proximal axon then begins to sprout new branches that cross the damaged area and attempt to grow into the distal empty tube. If they are successful in reaching the distal tube, they would continue to grow into the target organ to restore innnervation. The rate of growth is about 1 mm / day. If not, they sprout into the surrounding tissue or within the damaged epineureum to form a tangle called a neuroma.

In the muscle, the fibres tend to degenerate resulting in wasting of the muscle. There are changes in the EMG with denervation potentials and fibrillations seen after 10 - 14 days following injury. If innervation occurs before the muscle is completely wasted and replaced with fibrous tissue, return of function could be expected.

Classification of nerve injuries
Nerve injuries are classified depending on the extent. Seddon's classification introduced in 1943 identifies three stages.

a.) Neuropraxia is a transient functional impairment with no structural damage to the nerve.
b.) Axonotmesis is interruption of the axon with no disruption of the endoneurium so that the endoneureal tube remains in continuity. Thus regeneration could be complete with a potential for complete recovery.
c.) Neurotmesis is where the endoneureal tubes are disrupted and unless they are restored into continuity, recovery of function would be unlikely.

The Sunderland classification introduced more recently has 5 grades.

Grade I	Loss of axon conduction with no structural injury.
Grade II	Loss of axonal continuity with intact endoneureal tubes
Grade III	Loss of axonal and endoneureal continuity but intact perineureum
Grade IV	Loss of perineureal continuity and fascicular disruption but intact epineurium.
Grade V	Loss of continuity of entire nerve trunk.

Clinical features
Following injury to a peripheral nerve, there is impaired function in the region of distribution of that nerve. The functions disturbed are:
1. Motor function as evidenced by weakness or paralysis of muscles innervated by that nerve.
2. Sensory function as evidenced by loss of all forms of sensation in the area of distribution

of the nerve.
3. Autonomic function as evidenced by loss of sweating, piloerection and loss of vascular tone in the innervated region.
Electrophysiological studies help to confirm the injury.

Management

Management of patients with peripheral injuries is aimed at providing the best possible conditions for the nerve to regenerate and to maintain the target organs in an optimum condition for restoration of function when regeneration has been achieved.

Grade I injuries recover completely within a short period of time and do not require any special procedures other than reassurance of the patient.

Grade II injuries also recover completely but time has to be allowed for the nerve to regenerate. During this period, the muscles and joints should be maintained in an optimum position of function with regular physiotherapy.

Grade III to V injuries require surgical repair or neurorrhaphy. The nerve fascicles should be approximated as accurately as possible to enable the sprouting axons to reach the distal endoneurial tubes. This can be achieved by accurate epineurial repair where the entire nerve trunk is approximated end to end. or perineureal repair between each fascicle. Prior to repair, any neuroma has to be resected and the nerve ends divided to expose the growing axon sprouts proximally as well as the empty endoneurial tubes distally. The approximation must be without tension and where there is a large gap between the two ends, nerve grafts have to be used to bridge the gap. There is no clear evidence to indicate that interfasicular repair is superior to nerve trunk repair in terms of return of function. Following any form of nerve repair, successful outcome depends on physiotherapy to maintain the distal tissues in an optimum functional position.

Entrapment neuropathies

Entrapment neuropathy occurs either when a peripheral nerve is compressed during its course through a fibro-osseous tunnel or during its passage between two heads of a muscle. In the former instance, the nerve is compressed either due to swelling of the nerve beyond the limits of the space permitted in the tunnel or if the tunnel is narrowed due to any deformity of the bone, joint or fibrous tissue that form its boundaries. In the latter instance, compression occurs only with movement where the two portions of the muscle pinch the nerve each time they contract.

The common entrapment neuropathies are:

Upper limb

Carpal tunnel syndrome	Median nerve compression in carpal tunnel
Cubital tunnel syndrome	Ulnar nerve at elbow between the two heads of flex. carpi ulnaris.
Median nerve at elbow	Compression by ligament of Struthers or pronator teres.
Digital nerves	Intermetacarpal tunnel

Lower limb
Meralgia paraesthetica	Lateral femoral cutaneous nerve below inguinal ligament.
Common peroneal nerve	Between peroneous longus and tibia
Tarsal tunnel syndrome	Posterior peroneal nerve in posterior tarsal tunnel
Morton's syndrome	Interdigital nerve compressed by the metatarsal ligament.

Brachial plexus
Thoracic outlet syndrome	Lower trunk of the brachial plexus by the first rib or scalenus anterior.

Head
Occipital neuralgia	Occipital nerve near the superior nuchal line.
Trigeminal neuralgia	The trigeminal nerve is compressed distal from the brainstem

Clinical features
Entrapment neuropathy causes sensory and/or motor disturbances in the area of distribution of the involved. The early symptoms are pain and paraesthesiae. There could be sensory deficits in the area of innervation or weakness of muscles supplied by the nerve. If untreated, permanent damage to the nerve could result with loss of sensation and paralysis of the muscles involved.

Investigations
The nerve compression can be confirmed with electrophysiological studies.

Treatment
Surgical decompression of the nerve is required in most instances. This is achieved by division of the band of tissue compressing the nerve and enlarging the passage for the nerve.

Peripheral nerve compression

Compression of peripheral nerves could occur due to intrinsic tumours such as neurofibromas within the nerve or extrinsic tumours, fibrosis or scar tissue outside the nerve. Sometimes malignant tumours infiltrate the nerves resulting in local destruction of the nerve as seen in Pancoast's syndrome. Fibrosis and scar tissue is seen following irradiation, or soft tissue injury such as from missiles and other penetrating wounds.

Management
Management of this sort of nerve compression is difficult. Surgical management is aimed at decompressing the nerve by dissecting it away from the tumour or soft tissue (neurolysis). In case of intrinsic tumours, the tumours can usually be excised leaving the nerve in continuity. If the nerve is involved in the pathological process and cannot be decompressed, excision and grafting may become necessary.

Following any surgical procedure, recovery takes a long time depending on the rate of nerve regeneration and structured physiotherapy and rehabilitation aimed at maintaining optimum joint and muscle function is required during the interim period.

13

CONGENITAL ABNORMALITIES

Contents

Development of the central nervous system
Developmental abnormalities of the brain
Developmental abnormalities of the spine

Congenital abnormalities of the central nervous system could involve the cranium, spine or both.

Development of the central nervous system

The nervous system develops from the primitive neuroectoderm which originally is in the form of a plate. A ridge like thickening called the neural crest develops in the plate extending from the rostral to the caudal end. This ridge invaginates to form the neural groove which then detaches from the ectoderm to form the neural tube. The central nervous system develops from this neural tube. The rostral end after a series of foldings, develops into the brain and the caudal end to the spinal cord. Mesodermal tissue is then laid over the neural tube to for the skull and the vertebral column.

Some congenital anomalies such as anencephaly (absence of the brain) are incompatible with life while others such as spina bifida occulta may not cause any visible deformity or disability and go unnoticed. Some of the severe abnormalities could be detected in-utero on ultra sound scanning and the pregnancy may be terminated.

Developmental abnormalities of the brain

Common development abnormalities affecting the brain are hydrocephalus and craniosynostosis.

Hydrocephalus

Hydrocephalus results due to malformations in the arachnoid granulations that absorb CSF or due to malformations in the ventricular system. As CSF accumulates, the ventricular system dilates and the head enlarges. The cerebral cortex becomes thinned out. Despite this, most babies do not show any neurological disability.

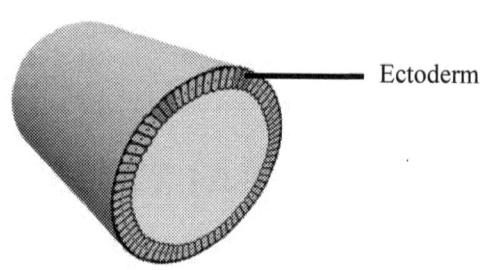
Ectoderm

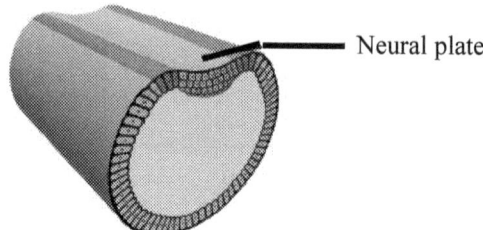
Neural plate

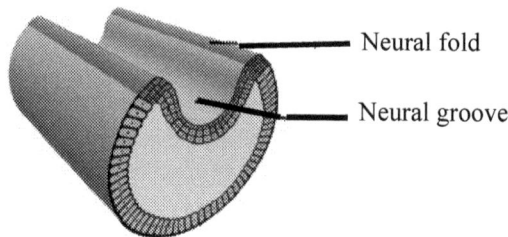
Neural fold
Neural groove

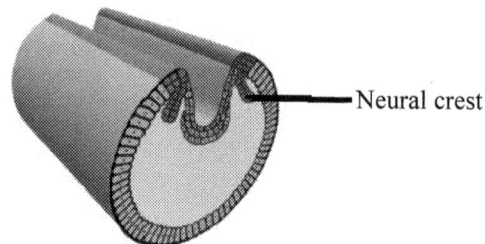
Neural crest

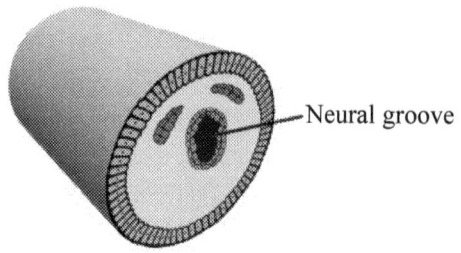
Neural groove

Clinical features

Hydrocephalus is evident as an increase in the skull circumference over the standard limits of maturity. The fontanel fails to close and there may be difficulty with upward gaze resulting in the eyes being turned downward and the cornea partially hidden by the lower lid (sun set sign). The extent of hydrocephalus is evident on a CT scan

Treatment

Most cases of hydrocephalus are self limiting but if the head continues to enlarge, a CSF shunt is indicated. The common shunt used is a ventriculo-peritoneal, or ventriculo-atrial shunt. A recently developed operation designed to create a communication between the third ventricle and the basal cisterns using an endoscope is sometimes used (endoscopic third ventriculostomy).

Craniosynostosis

This is a condition where the skull bones fuse prematurely so that the growing brain is restricted within the calvarium. This results in raised intracranial pressure. Often there are accompanying abnormalities of the face as well.

Treatment is designed to create an artificial fontanel and divide the prematurely fused sutures so that the brain can resume its normal growth.

Developmental abnormalities of the spinal cord

The common developmental abnormality affecting the spinal cord is spina-bifida. This results in failure of the mesodermal elements to enclose the neural tube, leaving a defect through which neural tissue tends to bulge out of the skin. There are different grades of spina-bifida depending on the extent to which mesoderm fails to encompass the neural tube.

The mildest variety involves a defect in the neural arch of the spine often noticed in X-rays of the spine taken for other reasons. The vertebral spine appears bifid with no external abnormalities evident (**spina bifida occulta**). Sometimes, a lipoma or tuft of hair overlies the bifid spine and occasionally the lipoma may extend into the spinal canal leading to neural compression and neurological deficits. A more extensive defect in the spinal arch leads to a defect in the neural arch where the meninges bulge out (**meningocoele**). A pure meningocoele where there are no nerve roots within is uncommon. More commonly, the bulging sac contains nerve roots (**meningo-myelocoele**) and depending on the extent of nerve involvement, there may be neurological deficits ranging from dysfunction of a few nerve roots to complete paraplegia with absent bowel or bladder function. The most severe form of spina bifida involves the neural tube being completely open to the outside. This is evident as a patch of granulation tissue through which CSF extrudes out (**myelocoele**). This leads to complete paraplegia with absent bladder and bowel function and often the babies succumb to meningitis. The treatment is designed to excise the sac and repair the defect so that further herniation is prevented.

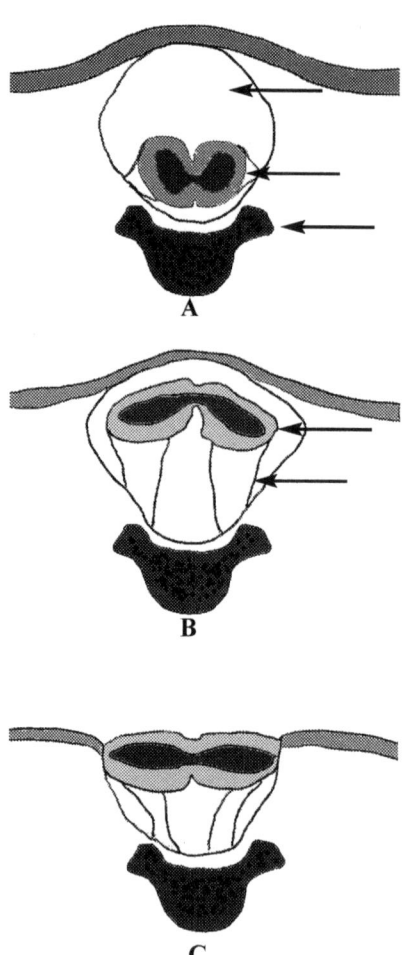

Figure 1. *A: Depicts a meningoele (top arrow), note how the spinal cord is normal (second arrow) and the third arrow demonstrates the associated spina bifida; B: This image depicts a myelomeningocoele. Note the unfolded placode (top arrow) covered by thinned and abnormal skin and how the nerve roots descend from the placode (bottom arrow); C: This image depicts myeloschisis. Note how the unfolded neural placode (arrow) is exposed to the air.*

14

INFECTION

Contents

Intracranial infections
Spinal Infections

Central nervous system infections may be either intracranial or spinal.

Intracranial infections

Intra cranial infections may involve the leptomeninges; pia and arachnoid resulting in meningitis or form abscesses. These abscesses could be epidural, subdural or intracerebral.

Spread of infection

Infection may spread into the intracranial cavity in different ways:

1. Direct implantation
Organisms could be directly implanted into the meninges or the brain parenchyma following penetrating injuries or due to open skull fractures where the meninges are torn and the brain lacerated. Direct implantation could also occur during surgery and with surgical implants such as ventricular shunts.

2. Direct spread
Direct intracranial spread of organisms may occur where the skull or the meninges are breached providing an avenue for infection. This could occur with open fractures of the skull vault or basal skull fractures open to the para nasal sinuses, pharynx or middle ear. Patients with CSF leak either through the nose, ear or pharynx are especially prone to intracranial spread of infection. Direct spread could also occur following neurosurgical procedures in post operative infection.

3. Spread from infection involving adjacent structures
Intracranial spread could occur from infections in adjacent structures such as the scalp, face, para nasal sinuses, middle ear and mastoid. Such infection could spread directly into the meninges or brain when the infective process causes destruction of the bone separating these structures from the intracranial cavity or when the infective process causes thrombosis of emissary veins communicating with intracranial veins. The thrombosed veins form an avenue for organisms to spread. In the event that the venous thrombosis causes devitalisation of the

brain parenchyma due to venous stasis and infarction, the resulting spread of infection could result in a brain abscess.

4. Blood stream spread
Organisms can be carried intracranially via the blood stream following septicemia or pyaemia. More commonly infected vegetations from cardiac valves can get detached and form septic embolii which are carried into the brain causing an infarction and formation of an abscess in the infarcted area. Such vegetations are common in cyanotic heart disease where the right to left shunt bypasses the lungs carrying the infection directly into the brain. Blood stream spread of infection is also seen in intravenous drug abusers.

Microbiology
The organisms responsible for CNS infections can be viruses, bacteria, fungi, protozoa and other parasites. Viral infections usually cause meningitis or encephalitis and do not require neurosurgical management. Bacterial infections could be acute due to stahylococci, streptococci, gram negative organisms such as E. coli and anaerobic organisms. Chronic bacterial infection is commonly due to tuberculosis. Fungal infections such as yeast or cryptococcus neoformans are more common in immunocompromised patients. Protozoal infections could occur with entamoeba histolytica which forms amoebic brain abscesses or as a complication of Falciparum malaria. Other parasitic infections are due to cysts from tape worms and cysticercosis.

Pathophysiology.
The pathophysiological alterations depend on the structures involved in the infection.

Meningitis
Acute bacterial meningitis results in irritation of the leptomeninges and leads to photophobia, neck stiffness and a positive Kernig's sign. There is also systemic evidence of an infection with fever and leucocytosis. In children, especially neonates, such infections could damage the arachnoid granulations resulting in communicating hydrocephalus. Also in neonates where the brain parenchyma is less mature, bacterial infections may result in permanent brain damage leading to epilepsy, mental retardation or cerebral palsy. Bacterial infections may also cause thrombosis of the cortical veins or the superior sagittal sinus resulting in venous infraction of the brain which could be fatal.

Chronic infections due to tuberculosis or fungi usually involve the base of the brain and basal adhesions could obstruct CSF flow resulting in a communicating hydrocephalus and raised ICP.
Chronic infections can also cause an endarteritis where blood supply to different regions of the brain could be impaired leading to infarction.

Epidural abscess
Epidural collection of pus commonly occurs following middle ear, mastoid or para nasal sinus infection or post operatively following infection of the bone flap. If the abscess is large there could be a mass effect with focal neurological signs and raised intra-cranial pressure. Otherwise, there would be only general signs of an infection or local signs where the skull over the abscess is often hyperaemic and swollen and may be tender.

Subdural abscess

Subdural abscess or empyema is often life threatening. The collection of pus in the subdural space may be extensive and cause brain displacement and raised intracranial pressure and focal neurological deficits. The infective process could also result in thrombosis of the cortical veins and venous infarction of the brain leading to permanent neurological disability.

Intracerebral abscess

Intracerebral abscess occurs within the brain parenchyma and could involve any part of the cerebral hemisphere or cerebellum. The abscess has a capsule which is thicker towards the outside where the rich blood supply from the pia results in a better fibrotic reaction. The wall tends to be thin towards the inside where the white matter is less vascular, and the fibrotic reaction not so pronounced. As such, when the abscess enlarges, it tends to extend into the white matter and bulge towards the ventricle and could ultimately rupture into the ventricle resulting in sudden death. The infective process in the abscess may lead to generalised symptoms such as headache, fever and feeling unwell and also cause a leucocytosis. The local involvement of the brain could result in focal neurological deficits. As the abscess enlarges, the mass effect could lead to brain displacement and raised ICP. Abscesses in the posterior cranial fossa may lead to compression of the fourth ventricle due to displacement of the cerebellum resulting in obstructive hydrocephalus.

Clinical Features

Patients with meningitis present with features of meningeal irritation such as headache, nausea, vomiting, neck stiffness and have a positive Kernig's sign. They also have features of an infection such as fever, malaise and rapidly become unwell. They often have a leucocytosis and raised ESR and CRP. Complications such as hydrocephalus may result in raised intracranial pressure which manifests as papilloedema and alteration of level of consciousness. If the cortical veins become thrombosed, they may develop epileptic seizures and focal neurological deficits. Thrombosis of the venous sinuses could cause raised ICP with papilloedema and altered consciousness and also lead to focal neurological deficits.

Those with intracranial suppuration present with features of raised ICP such as headache, vomiting and papilloedema together with features of systemic infection. If the abscess involves eloquent areas of the brain, focal neurological signs become manifest. Abscesses in the posterior cranial fossa could obstruct the fourth ventricle resulting in obstructive hydrocephalus and raised ICP.

Investigations

Investigations are designed to establish the diagnosis, determine the site of infection within the intracranial cavity, any complication and the microbiology of the infecting agent. A CT scan with contrast enhancement often shows the formation of an abscess and the anatomical plane of suppuration. Epidural abscess shows as a crescentic area of low density with enhancement of the dura. With subdural empyema, often CT abnormalities are slight, in contrast to the clinical condition, and subdural empyema is a frequent "missed diagnosis". Sometimes a more extensive area of low density is evident with enhancement of the capsule. Intracerebral abscesses appear as a well circumscribed area of low density with an enhancing capsule and a surrounding area of low density due to vasogenic oedema of the brain parenchyma. Hydrocephalus may be seen due to obstruction to CSF flow in cerebellar abscesses and also following basal adhesions in tuberculous or fungal meningitis. CT scans also reveal areas of venous or arterial infarction.

Peripheral blood examination reveals leucocytosis, raised ESR and CRP. Blood culture is essential to exclude a septicemia or bacteraemia. Where indicated, investigations should also be carried out to determine a possible focus of infection or evidence of immunosuppression. Microbiological investigations are carried out on peripheral blood, pus from an area of suppuration and CSF in cases of meningitis to determine the infecting agent and also the antibiotic sensitivity.

Treatment
Appropriate antibiotic treatment after isolation of the organism and its antibiotic sensitivity forms the mainstay of treatment. Uncomplicated meningitis is mainly managed with antibiotic treatment. In the event of complications such as hydrocephalus surgical drainage of the CSF would become necessary. This can be achieved either via a ventriculostomy or a ventriculo-peritoneal shunt.
Epidural abscess requires evacuation and micro biological analysis of the pus. This could be achieved via a burr hole. If the overlying skull shows evidence of osteomyelitis such as in infected bone flaps, the involved bone has also to be removed.
Subdural empyema is also treated with burr hole evacuation but sometimes could be difficult to treat and may require multiple burr holes for drainage with irrigation of the infected space with antibiotics.
Intracerebral abscess could be aspirated via a burr hole and with appropriate antibiotic treatment, the infection resolves. The progress of the abscess is followed up with repeated CT scans. If the abscess fails to respond to aspiration or if there are multiple loculii, excision of the capsule may become necessary. If the abscess is small, aspiration is carried out with stereotactic guidance.

Spinal Infections
Spinal infections usually form abscesses which could be epidural, subdural or intramedullary.

Spread of infection

Infection could spread into the spinal canal in different ways
1. Direct implantation
Organisms could be directly implanted into the spine following penetrating injuries such as stab wounds or missile injuries. Direct implantation could also occur during lumbar puncture, spinal operations and with surgical implants such as intra spinal catheters used for drug delivery or CSF drainage, stimulating electrodes such as in dorsal column stimulators and following spinal subarachnoid shunts.

2. Direct spread
Direct intra spinal spread of organisms commonly follows infection of the spine but could also occur from retro pharyngeal abscesses, mediastinal infections and retro peritoneal infections.

3. Spread from infection involving adjacent structures
Intra spinal spread could occur from infections in adjacent structures such as the pharynx, mediastinum, pleural cavity, retro peritoneal space, kidneys and pelvis. Such infection could spread directly into the spinal canal or via the para vertebral plexus.

4. Blood stream spread
Blood stream spread is the most common and usually takes place via the para vertebral plexus, or less commonly the systemic circulation.

Microbiology
The organisms responsible for spinal infection are similar to those involved in intracranial infection.

Pathophysiology.
The pathophysiological alterations depend on the structures involved in the infection.

Epidural abscess
Epidural collection of pus could be spontaneous or iatrogenic following surgery, epidural catheters or implants such as stimulators. Sometimes the patients are very ill and the infection is rapidly progressive leading to septicemia. In addition to the mass effect of the abscess and mechanical compression of the spinal cord, there is often a vascular element due to thrombosis of spinal arteries and veins leading to infarction of the spinal cord and paraplegia. There are general signs of an infection such as pyrexia and also local signs where the spine over the abscess is often tender. In the event of destruction and collapse of the vertebral body, there may be a kyphotic deformity.
Epidural abscess secondary to tuberculosis could be silent with no generalised evidence of an infection. Clinical manifestations may appear late with collapse of the vertebral body leading to a kyphotic deformity and spinal cord dysfunction (Pott's disease)

Subdural abscess
Subdural abscess of the spine is similar to the epidural abscess in its pathology.

Intramedullary abscess
Intramedullary abscess occurs within the spinal cord. There is compression of the white matter tracts with resulting spinal cord dysfunction leading to sensory, motor and autonomic changes below the level of the lesion. The infective process in the abscess may also lead to generalised symptoms such as fever and feeling unwell and also cause a leucocytosis.

Clinical Features
Patients with spinal infection present with features of spinal cord compression such as sensory, motor and autonomic disturbances below the level of the lesion. They also have features of an infection such as fever, malaise and rapidly become unwell. They often have a leucocytosis and raised ESR and CRP. If the spinal blood vessels become thrombosed, they develop paraplegia or quadruplegia which could be permanent.

Investigations
Investigations are designed to establish the diagnosis, determine the site of infection within the spinal canal and the microbiology of the infecting agent. A MRI scan with contrast enhancement is the most useful and shows the formation of the abscess and the anatomical plane and extent of suppuration within the spinal canal as well as the para spinal tissues. Changes of signal within the spinal cord may indicate spinal ischaemia.
Peripheral blood examination reveals leucocytosis, raised ESR and CRP. Blood culture is essential to exclude a septicemia or bacteraemia. Where indicated, investigations should also

be carried out to determine a possible focus of infection or evidence of immunosuppresion. Microbiological investigations are carried out on peripheral blood an pus from an area of suppuration. Histological examination of material removed at surgery are also useful is tuberculous and fungal infections.

Treatment
Treatment is aimed at decompressing the spinal cord and appropriate antibiotic treatment after isolation of the organism and establishing its antibiotic sensitivity. This is carried out via a laminectomy. Stabilisation procedures may be necessary in cases where the spine is unstable due to destruction of the vertebral bodies by the disease process. The neurological sequelae could be long standing or permanent resulting in paraplegia and following the period of acute treatment, a comprehensive program of rehabilitation may be required.

15

ICU MANAGEMENT

Contents

Raised intracranial pressure (ICP)
Monitoring
  Intracranial pressure monitoring
  Measurement of cerebral blood flow
  EEG and Bispectral analysis (BIS)
  Brain tissue oxygen tension monitoring ($PbtO_2$)
The injured brain
  Management of ICP and CPP in brain injury
  Brain herniation
Status epilepticus

Raised intracranial pressure (ICP)

Pathophysiology of raised ICP

The pathophysiology of raised ICP due for example to a space occupying lesion (SOL) is based on the notion that the skull vault in an adult is nearly indistensible and the contents within nearly incompressible. However, both CSF and blood could be displaced from the vault and the brain could displace within the vault from one compartment to another. As such, when a SOL expands within the skull, initially the space required for the SOL will be provided by CSF leaving the intracranial cavity and later to some extent by a reduction in blood volume. Thus, the total volume of the intracranial contents are unchanged and there is hardly any change in ICP. However, when all the available CSF and blood has been displaced, the near incompressibility of the intracranial contents cause a rapid increase in ICP due to very small further increments in volume of the SOL. (Monroe Kellie Doctrine). The brain which is displaced by the SOL herniates under the falx to the opposite side (sub falcine herniation), through the tentorial hiatus towards the posterior cranial fossa (trans tentorial herniation) and the cerebellar tonsils tends to herniate through the foramen magnum towards the spinal canal (tonsillar herniation)

Clinical features of raised ICP

As the ICP increases, the patient develops symptoms such as headache, vomiting and also papilloedema in long standing cases. (Papilloedema may occur as soon as six hours after developing an SOL). As the ICP continues to increase functional disturbances occur. There will be difficulty in maintaining cerebral perfusion due to a tendency towards a fall in cerebral perfusion pressure (CPP). (CPP = Mean art. BP - ICP)

In order to maintain an adequate CPP, the systemic BP increases and to ensure a forceful expulsion of blood into the intra-cranial cavity, the diastolic filling time of the heart increases thereby causing a bradycardia. The respiratory rate also tends to increase so that the increase in ICP is reflected as changes of vital signs. The classical change with raised ICP is a falling pulse rate and a rising blood pressure.

As the brain herniates, there is distortion of the brain stem that results in impaired consciousness recognised as a drop in the GCS score. The herniating brain also compresses the IIIrd cranial nerves, initially on the side of the lesion causing an ipsilateral pupillary dilatation and later bilateral pupillary dilatation. Sometimes a complete IIIrd nerve palsy may be seen with ptosis and lateral deviation of the eye. Brain displacement also causes focal neurological deficits to appear depending on the site of the expanding lesion.

In summary, the functional changes due to raised ICP consist of
1. Changes in vital signs, falling pulse rate and increasing blood pressure
2. Drop in GCS score
3. Ipsilateral pupillary dilatation followed by bilateral involvement
4. Focal neurological signs depending on the site of the lesion.

The functional changes with rise of ICP are reversible if the SOL or causative factor is removed. However, if untreated ICP will continue to increase and result in a secondary haemorrhage into the brain stem. If such an event occurs subsequent removal of the SOL will have no benefit of complete recovery due to the secondary damage caused to the brain stem. Secondary brain stem haemorrhage results in a reversal of the cardio-vascular response (also called the Cushing's response) where the pulse rate now increases and the BP falls accompanied by Cheyne-Stokes respiration and also hyper-pyrexia due to impaired temperature regulation. The patient has a GCS of 3, bilateral fixed and dilated pupils and a decerebrate posture following which death usually ensues.

Management of raised ICP
Management of patients where raised ICP is envisaged consists of
1. Observing for functional changes outlined above.
2. Diagnosis of cause of ICP
3. Definitive treatment of ICP depending on cause.

Tonsillar herniation could irritate the first cervical nerves that supply the sub occipital muscles causing these muscles to contract resulting in neck stiffness. This could be easily mistaken for meningism and prompt one to undertake a lumbar puncture. This would have disastrous consequences as the release of CSF from the spinal theca will facilitate further tonsillar herniation around the medulla leading to coning and instant death.

Monitoring

Intracranial pressure monitoring
Measurements are currently performed invasively. Devices are either catheter based or non-catheter based. In catheter based systems the intracranial pressure is measured with the aid of an external ventricular drain. This can either be done by transducing/measuring the height of the fluid column of the catheter or by incorporating a solid state/fibre optic transducer within the catheter. Non-catheter based systems are solid state/fibre optic transducers that are

left intracranially at the time of surgery or inserted via a twist drill and bolt system. The transducer tip can either be placed subdurally or in the parenchyma of the brain. The most reliable way and the gold standard for intracranial pressure monitoring is intraventricular pressure monitoring via an external ventricular drain. The ICP readings are the most accurate reflection of intracranial pressure of any of the systems and intracranial hypertension may be treated by CSF drainage. Transducers in the parenchyma and those located subdurally can only account for the pressures of the parenchyma directly adjacent to the sensor. The advantage of the non catheter based systems is that they have a lower infectious potential. The *Codman* system is a silicon chip solid state system and the *Camino* system a fibre optic system.

The ICP is measured continuously via a monitor and a wave pattern is seen. The normal wave demonstrates slow fluctuations due to respiration with superimposed biphasic cardiac generated fluctuations. Usually the cardiac fluctuations are relatively small compared to the respiratory fluctuations. These can be imagined as large ocean waves (respiratory waves) with ripples on them (cardiac oscillations). In cases of reduced brain compliance the cardiac fluctuations become more pronounced.

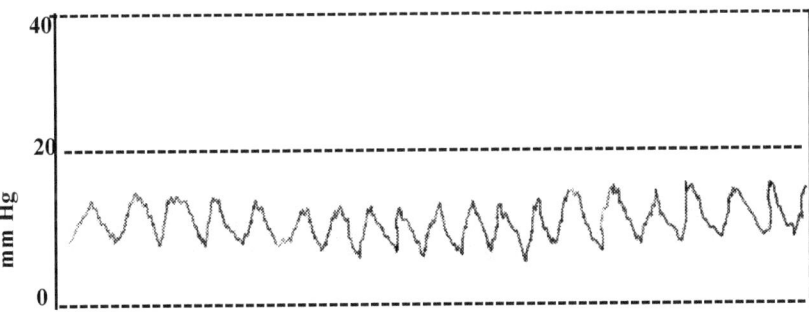

Figure 1 - *The normal ICP breathing curve.*

Reduced compliance and elevated ICP can lead to pathological waves as described by Lundberg:

Lundberg A (plateau waves) - These waves have a continued increase in the baseline ICP of 50 mm Hg or more and have a duration of 5 – 20 minutes. When they terminate, the baseline ICP is reset to a higher value. These waves are a poor prognostic sign and indicate that there is severely reduced intracranial compliance.

Lundberg B waves - These are less severe, last for 2 minutes or less and have lower amplitudes than A waves, and are commonly in the region of 10-20 mm Hg. They may be either sinus-like or ramp-like.

Lundberg C waves (Herring-Traube-Mayer waves) - These are of very limited pathological significance and are caused mainly by physiological fluctuations with low amplitudes and can be superimposed on the normal pattern.

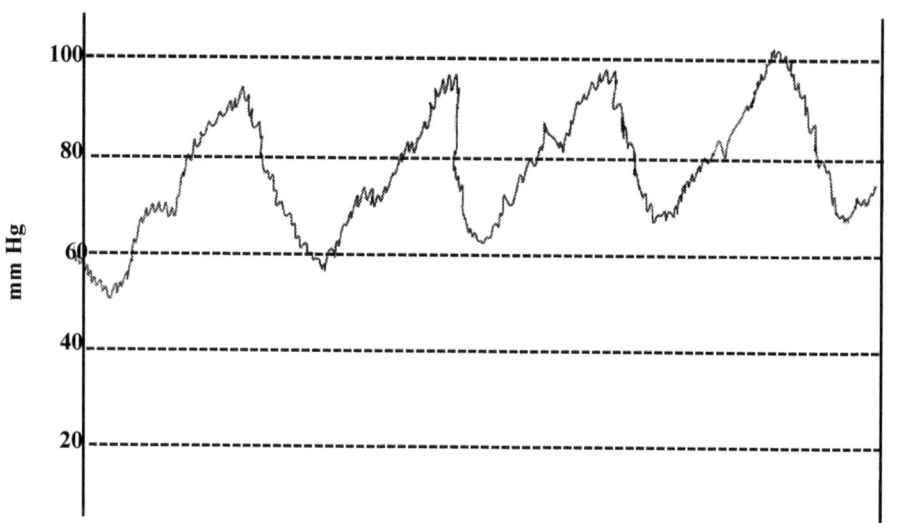

Figure 2 - *Lundberg A wave. These waves have a continued increase in the baseline ICP of 50 mm Hg or more and have a duration of 5 – 20 minutes.*

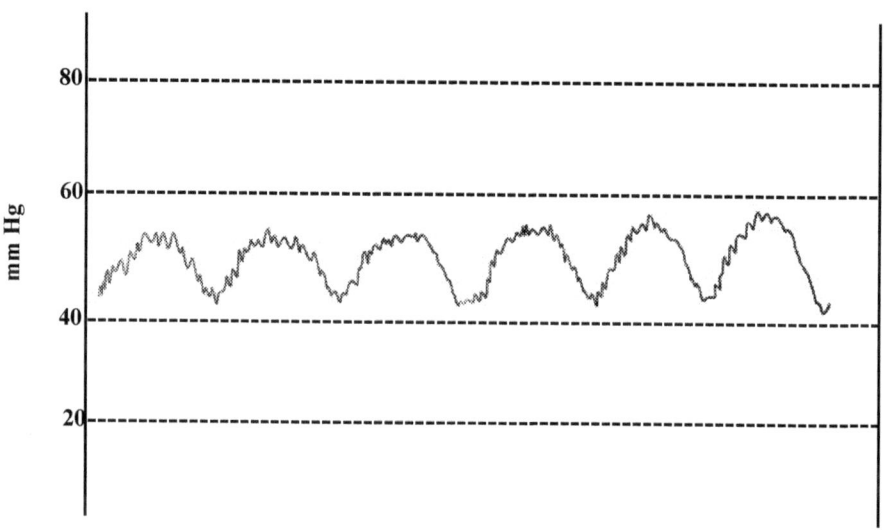

Figure 3. *Sinus-like B-waves. These are independent of changes of blood pressure, breathing, or CO_2 level.*

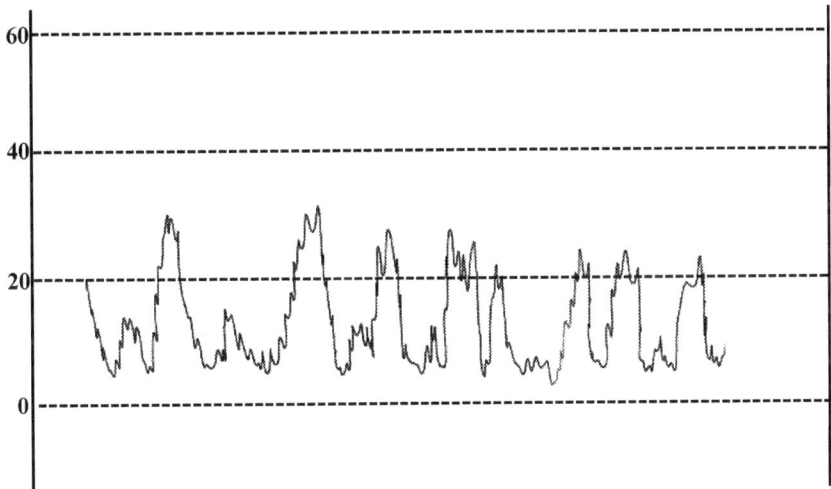

Figure 4. *Ramp-like B-waves. These are produced by snoring and concomitant pCO_2 increases*

Measurement of cerebral blood flow

Transcranial Doppler Ultrasonography (TCD)

This is a non invasive method to indirectly measure the blood flow by measuring the velocity of intracranial blood flow. This is done by monitoring the shift in frequency spectra of the Doppler signal. By using a 2 MHz probe and using the natural windows to the intracranial space, the temporal bone, orbital foramen and the foramen magnum, signals are obtained that have proven to be clinically useful. The most common route is to measure the middle cerebral artery through the temporal bone. There is a proportional change in velocity and blood flow if the diameter of the blood vessel stays unchanged. A rise in flow velocity means that either the blood flow has increased or that the vessel diameter has decreased. To be able to tell whether a patient is hyperaemic or has vasospasm, the hemispheric index is used. This is the flow velocity of the middle cerebral artery divided by the flow velocity of the ipsilateral extracranial internal carotid artery. A value of greater than 3 indicates vasospasm. TCD is useful for monitoring CBF non invasively, diagnosing vasospasm and monitoring the response of treatment of vasospasm.

Jugular Venous Oximetry (JVO)

This is an indirect measurement of the cerebral blood flow (CBF) based on the fact that the cerebral metabolic rate of oxygen ($CMRO_2$) is equal to the CBF multiplied by the difference in the arterial and venous oxygen concentration ((A-V)DO2)

$$CMRO_2 = CBF \times (A-V)DO_2.$$

Both the cerebral arterial oxygenation and the CMRO2 is usually constant, therefore any decrease in the venous oxygen saturation is usually an indication that the blood flow is reduced and that the tissue is extracting more oxygen out of the slow flowing blood. The measurement is done with a catheter placed in a retrograde fashion into the jugular bulb via the internal jugular vein. The tip of the catheter must be in or within 1 cm of the bulb to stop the blood from becoming mixed with extracranial blood. Three indices can be obtained from JVO monitoring:

$SVJO_2$ (The saturation of the JVO)
A normal value is between 60-80%, and a value of 90% or more indicates hyperemia, and a value of 50% or less, indicates hypoperfusion (there is very little time for oxygen to be extracted from fast flowing blood).

CEO_2 (The cerebral oxygen extraction)
This is the difference between the arterial and jugular venous oxygen content. A normal value is between 24% and 40% with values lower than this range indicating hyperemia and higher values indicating hypoperfusion (there is a higher extraction of oxygen in slow flowing blood).

(A-V)DO_2 (The difference in the arterial and venous oxygen concentration)
Normal values are 5-7.5 vol % and lower values indicate hyperemia and higher values hypoperfusion.

Therefore a high $SVJO_2$ with low CEO_2 and (A-V) DO_2 indicates hyperemia and vice versa. It has been proven with the aid of JVO monitoring that patients suffer from episodes of decreased cerebral perfusion despite and adequate cerebral perfusion pressure. There is good outcome in patients who have JVO monitoring. The criticism of JVO monitoring is that it only supplies a global picture of brain perfusion and cannot identify focal areas of ischaemia.

Near infrared spectroscopy (NIRS)
This is a non invasive method for measuring regional blood flow. Light in the near infrared range can penetrate skin, bone and soft tissue up to a depth of 8cm and is absorbed at different spectra by oxygenated haemoglobin, deoxygenated haemoglobin and cytochrome aa_3. Changes in absorption can be measured and in infants this is done with transillumination and in adults it is measured from reflected light due to the thickness of the skull. Different equations can derive measurements for regional blood flow, cerebral oxygen saturation, cerebral metabolism and cerebral blood volume. In the clinical setting this technology is still hampered by the confounding effects of extracranial blood flow. Intracranial haematomas also skew measurements. A cerebral oxygen saturation of higher than 75% suggests adequate CPP and values lower than 55% suggest inadequate CPP. Current clinical experience has proven that, in adults, cerebral blood flow and cerebral blood volume are significantly underestimated. It may prove a very useful tool in the future.

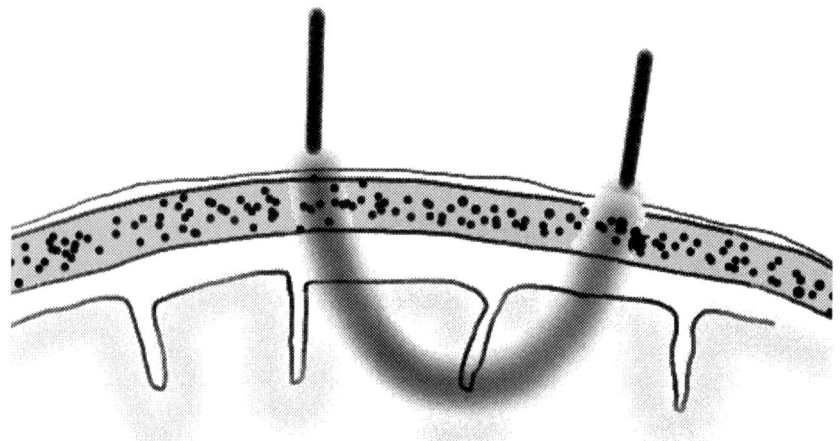

Figure 4. *Near infrared spectroscopy. The beam traverses the skull and soft tissue and is measured by the receiving probe.*

EEG and Bispectral analysis (BIS)

This is a tool that us used in both theatre and ICU to monitor the level of anaesthesia. Automated EEG processing has allowed bispectral analysis to become possible. A combination of different EEG processing parameters, obtained from a monitoring electrode strip with adhesive backing placed on the forehead, are used to make up the bispectral analysis. The bispectral index has been developed from a large amount of EEG data gathered from both volunteers and patients under different levels of sedation and ranges from a numerical value of 0 to 100. A value of 100 means that there is no sedation, 70 indicates a light hypnotic state, 60 indicates a moderate hypnotic state, 40 indicates a deep hypnotic state and 0 indicated EEG suppression. This value has been established in patients without brain damage and its use in patients with head injury is not validated. It is also important to realise that electromyogenic activity will give a falsely high number and therefore non paralysed patients could be over sedated. This is also true for the new BIS*xp* monitor.

Brain tissue oxygen tension monitoring ($PbtO_2$)

Direct regional measurements of the oxygenation of brain tissue can be performed using miniature Clarke's electrodes. There are two skull bolt systems currently available, the *Licox* system that measures brain tissue oxygen tension and temperature and the *Neurotrend* monitor that measures brain tissue oxygen tension, carbon dioxide tension, pH and temperature. The *Licox* device has two separate probes with sensors and the *Neurotrend* has one probe with four different sensors arranged along its 2 cm length. Normal values for $PbtO_2$ are 20-40 mmHg and there is increased risk of death for any period that the value is below 15 mmHg. Jugular venous oxygen monitoring correlates well with brain tissue oxygen tension monitoring and a $SVJO_2$ value of 50% correlates with a $PbtO_2$ value of 8.5 mm Hg. A combination of the global measurement of $SVJO_2$ and the local measurement of $PbtO_2$ is useful in the management of patients with brain injury.

Microdialysis

This is an invasive direct monitoring modality for the substrate and metabolites of the brain and is used to measure glucose, lactate, pyruvate, neurotransmitters and the levels of therapeutic agents. The catheter is very fine with a diameter of 0.5 mm and is perfused by a physiological solution at low flow rates. This is still mostly used for research activities and is quite labour intensive.

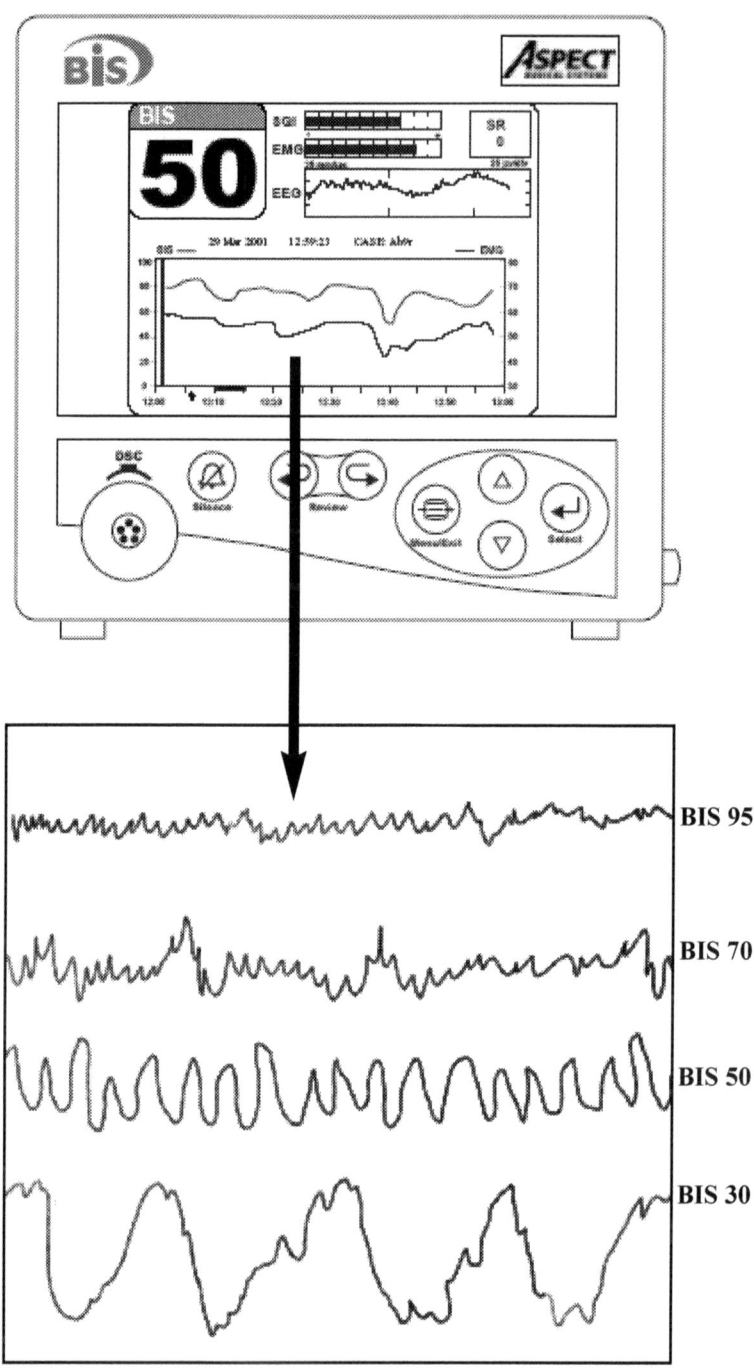

Figure 5. *The BIS monitor. See legend on opposite page.*

Figure 5. *The BIS monitor. See image on opposite page. There are several indices that are displayed on the monitor. The BIS value is indicated in the top left hand corner. In the right hand corner, the following 3 indices are displayed:* **The Signal Quality Index (SQI)** *Bar Graph is an indication of the quality of the EEG signal and optimal signal quality is indicated when the bar extends to the right side (+) of the graph.* **The Electromyograph (EMG)** *Bar Graph shows muscle activity. A low level of EMG is indicated when the bar is not present or at the left side of the graph.* **The Suppression Ratio (SR)** *Number is a calculated parameter to indicate when an isoelectric (flatline) condition may exist. Suppression ratio is the percentage of time over the last 63-second period that the signal is considered to be in the suppressed state. For example: SR=23 (isoelectric over 23% of the last 63 second review). The SR is displayed in the upper right corner of the screen. .*
The Electroencephalogram (EEG) Waveform Display is also on the top right-hand side. The main monitor demonstrates the trend. The bottom figure on the opposite page demonstrates the EEG slowing seen in progressively lower BIS values.

Evoked potentials

These potentials are generated by external stimulation of the nervous system and the potentials generated are then recorded. These potentials are much smaller that the normal background electrical activity and therefore a large number of impulses are generated and they are then averaged to account for the background noise. There are two basic types of evoked potential, sensory and motor.

Sensory evoked potentials – these are brainstem auditory evoked potentials (BAEP) which are generated by stimulating the eighth cranial nerve and recording the response by brainstem nuclei; visual evoked potentials (VEP) which is the response of the occipital cortex to visual stimulation by diodes during surgery and somatosensory evoked potentials (SSEP) which is the brain and spinal cord's response to the stimulation of a peripheral nerve. In the lower limb it is usually the posterior tibial nerve and in the upper limb it is usually the median or ulnar nerve.

Motor evoked potentials (MEP) – These are generated by transcranial stimulation of the cortex and the impulses can be measured in the epidural space, the peripheral nerves or in the muscles.

BAEP is used in surgery of the cerebellopontine angle, VEP is used for surgery around the optic nerves and optic chiasm and SSEP and MEP are used for spinal surgery.

The injured brain

Whatever kind of injury the brain receives, it is essential that the brain tissue is properly perfused. The cells of the brain do not have the capacity to store energy and if they are not constantly perfused, they die. When they die, the patient dies. The brain cannot be perfused if the blood pressure is too low for blood to flow through the brain or if the pressure is too high inside the cranium for blood to be able to flow through it. Therefore management of intracranial pressure and cerebral perfusion pressure is central to the management of the patient with brain injury.

ICP and CPP

The Monroe – Kelly doctrine is central to understanding the pathophysiology of raised intracranial pressure, compliance and elastance. It states that the fixed space contained within the skull is composed of brain, CSF and the blood contained in the vascular system. If either one of these increases then it does so to the detriment of the other two. An intracranial mass lesion has a deleterious effect on all three components. The two concepts that describe the effects of the Monroe - Kelly doctrine are elastance and compliance.

Intracranial elastance is the change in intracranial pressure as a function of a change of volume.

Intracranial compliance is the change in volume as a function as a function of the change in pressure.

Elastance describes the effect that added intracranial volume will have on the intracranial pressure. The elastance as can be seen from the elastance curve is the change in pressure over the change in volume or dP/dV. As elastance increases, a smaller change in volume results in the same amount of change in pressure. Compliance is exactly the opposite of that and is the change in volume due to a change in pressure or dV/dP. The practical effect of increased elastance is that intracranial haematomas, oedema, hyperemia, hydrocephalus and tumours increase the intracranial pressure to a critical level. There is capacity for the brain to accommodate some increased volume by displacing CSF up to a point. After this the pressure increases dramatically for a very small increase in volume.

The reason that a raised ICP has a deleterious effect on the brain is that it has a negative effect on the cerebral perfusion pressure (CPP). The equation that demonstrates the relationship between mean blood pressure (MAP), ICP and CPP is as follows: CPP = MAP – ICP.

The cerebral vasculature has the ability to autoregulate the blood flow by vasoconstriction and vasodilatation. This is intact for MAP's between 50 mmHg and 140 mmHg. Outside of these values autoregulation cannot function and the relation between blood flow and MAP becomes linear. In brain injured patients the autoregulation mechanism is frequently dysfunctional and the linear relationship takes over. When the relationship between MAP and blood flow becomes linear a drop in the MAP leads to a drop in the intracerebral blood flow and vice versa. If blood flow falls below a certain level, brain cell ischaemia follows and if the levels are low enough, there is failure of the transmembrane pumps and the associated influx of calcium leads to cell death. It is known that in patients with head injury the outcome is significantly worse if the CPP falls to below 60 mmHg. When CPP falls below 40 mmHg, a vasopressor response increases the MAP through a massive release of catecholamines, This is called the Cushing response which is typified by an increase in the systemic blood pressure and if there is associated central herniation (coning), bradycardia.

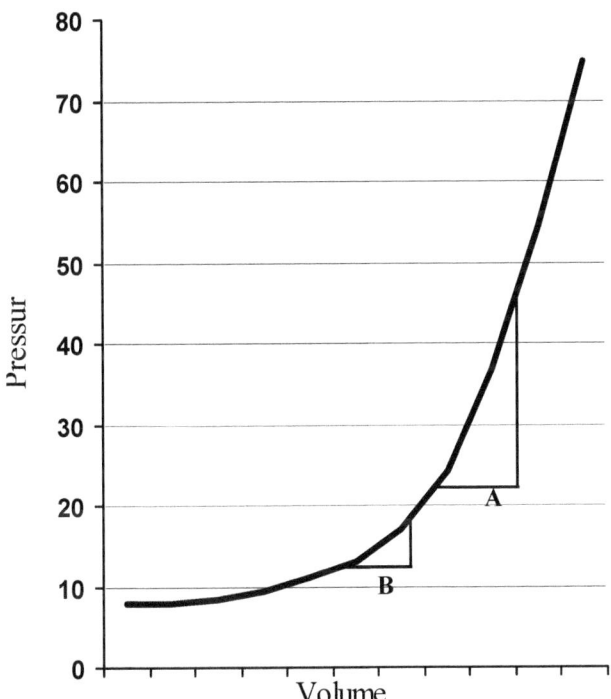

Figure 6. *The elastance curve. The elastance as can be seen from the curve is the change in pressure over the change in volume or dP/dV. Note that on the steeper part of the curve (A) , a small increase in volume, leads to a greater increase in pressure compared to on the less steep part of the curve (B).*

Management of ICP and CPP in brain injury
Medical therapy
Primary principles
The aim is to perfuse the brain (with well oxygenated blood containing the right concentration of glucose) by increasing the CPP to above 70 mmHg (some say 60 or 65 is acceptable) by either decreasing the ICP, increasing the MAP or both. An ICP consistently above 25 mmHg (some say 20 mmHg) is the threshold that requires treatment.

Position
Placing patients in a 10 – 15% head up position assists in venous drainage and helps to lower the ICP.

Ventilation
Normoventilation or slight hyperventilation is the current approach. Hyperventilation was used previously as it was though that the lowered $PaCO_2$ would lead to beneficial vasoconstriction with subsequent decreased ICP (Monroe – Kelly). However this lead to ischaemia in brain tissue already starved of perfusion. Keeping the $PaCO_2$ around 4.5 kPa or slightly lower is the current approach. Short periods of hyperventilation with FiO_2 of 100% can be used in conjunction with mannitol for sudden acute rises in ICP such as patients with traumatic extra axial collections on their way to theatre.

Temperature
It is important to maintain normothermia. Hyperthermia leads to increased metabolic work and subsequent increases in ICP. It was thought that hypothermia might decrease the ICP and have a neuroprotective effect. No definite benefit of induced hypothermia was found in

adults and increased infection, coagulopathy and arrhythmias have complicated this treatment. There is thought to be some benefit in children.

Electrolytes
Sodium is the most important electrolyte for the neurosurgeon and neurosurgical intensivist.

Hyponatremia leads to brain swelling and lowers the seizure threshold. Hyponatremia is frequently found in SAH. It is associated with high volume infusions of sodium poor fluids, cerebral salt wasting (CSW) and the syndrome of inappropriate ADH secretion (SIADH). It can be difficult to discern between SIADH and CSW. Both these conditions lead to low serum sodium, CSW does so because there is a loss of salt and SIADH does so because of water intoxication. In SIADH vasopressin is secreted despite volume overload. A low CVP or pulmonary capillary wedge pressure (PCWP) with increased hematocrit is typical of CSW. As a broad distinction, cases with CSW are dehydrated, and cases with SIADH are fluid overloaded (water intoxication). It is important to distinguish between these two as the treatment for CSW is fluid and sodium replacement which can be fatal in cases of SIADH. Conversely the treatment of SIADH is fluid restriction which can be fatal in cases of CSW, especially when occurring in SAH.

Hypernatremia may lead to restlessness, confusion and coma. It may be caused by over zealous administration of normal saline. Another more sinister cause is diabetes insipidus (DI) due to insufficient vasopressin (ADH) which leads to large amounts of fluid and electrolytes being lost as urine output dramatically increases. Central DI may be caused by any damage to the hypophysis or hypothalamus following transsphenoidal surgery, trauma, vascular infarct and compression from sellar tumours. The diagnosis is made by noting large volumes of dilute urine, more than 250 ml/hr in three consecutive hours with a low specific gravity (S.G) in the range of 1.001 to 1.005. Care must be taken not to confuse this with the patient who is having a diuresis due to a large fluid load. This is frequently seen in patients returning from theatre that have had large amounts of fluid infused. It is always helpful to look at the total fluid balance. In cases of DI the large urine output will be associated with raised serum osmolality and serum sodium. The urine will also be dilute macroscopically. Treatment is with desmopressin and fluid replacement. In the awake patient oral intake may be all that is required but in the comatose patient IV fluid needs to be infused or water may be given via the nasogastric route. It is important to use sodium-poor fluid and also to restrict dietary intake of sodium by low-sodium diet or nasogastric feed. DI may be temporary or permanent.

Magnesium has neuroprotective qualities and should be supplemented if levels are low.
Glucose control and nutrition
Hyperglycemia leads to lactate build up which mediates cell damage. Hypoglycemia leads to energy failure of the cells. It is imperative that patients are on a very tight glucose control and all patients should be on an insulin sliding scale. Feeding should be instituted as early as possibly, preferably within 24 – 48 hours to provide for both the energy needs of the injured brain and also to combat stress ulcers. The patient with an injured brain needs 1.5 times the normal amount of calories. H_2 receptor antagonists, proton pump inhibitors or sucralfate should also be used to combat stress ulcers.
Seizures
Phenytoin is effective in reducing early seizures, although it has no effect on the long term development of epilepsy. Convulsions increase the metabolic activity of the brain and may also cause muscle activity which can increase the ICP. Both Phenytoin and Phenobarbitone can be loaded IV and are effective in terminating seizures.
Blood pressure
Adequate MAP prevents reflex intracranial vasodilatation with resultant hyperemia as part of cerebral autoregulation when autoregulation is intact. When autoregulation is intact an ade-

quate MAP leads to an adequate CPP. When the autoregulation is not functioning, a MAP that is too high will lead to intracranial hyperemia. To sustain the MAP, adequate intravascular filling and the use of inotropic support, when the blood pressure is still low despite adequate filling, is used. When the systolic pressure rises above 200 -210 mmHg, this may lead to intracranial haemorrhage. Control of blood pressure should be done carefully as a sudden drop of filling pressure in cases where the brain is already ischemic, may lead to infarction. Therefore a short acting agent that can be titrated is recommended. Labetalol is a short acting beta blocker which is frequently used and titrated as an IV infusion.

Hyperosmolar therapy
Mannitol is an osmotically active compound that is used as the mainstay of treatment of raised ICP. It acts by osmotically drawing fluid from the brain parenchyma and excreting this fluid as part of a general osmotic diuresis. It also has the properties of being able to decreases CSF production; lowers blood viscosity and leads to improved rheology; it reduces brain swelling and oedema and is a free radical scavenger. It is usually used in 0.25g/kg boluses. Serum osmolality should be kept below 320 mosmol. It may be administered in conjunction with, and is potentiated by, loop diuretics (frusemide). Mannitol however can have a detrimental effect on patients with raised ICP secondary to hyperemia due to its effect on rheology. Hypertonic saline is being evaluated currently as a promising new treatment modality to reduce ICP and improve intracranial blood flow.

Sedation
Patients should always be deeply sedated to control ICP. Agents that are commonly used are propofol, fentanyl and midazolam. Propofol is used as an infusion and has the advantage that it does not accumulate and has a very short wash out period. Consequently patients can be roused very quickly following cessation of propofol infusion. It is also a very potent agent and can be used to provide burst suppression in salvage ICP management and intractable epilepsy.

Ventriculostomy
Draining CSF through an external ventricular drain is the most effective way of controlling the ICP. Drains are commonly set at the level of pressure that is acceptable or desired and any rises above that pressure will then produce CSF drainage and reduce the ICP (Monroe – Kelly). The zero mark is usually set at the external auditory meatus and the reservoir at 10 or 15 mmHg.

Neuromuscular blockade
Atracurium is non cumulative, not associated with myopathy and is commonly used in the intensive care to paralyse patients to reduce the ICP by reducing movement, coughing and straining and decrease muscle tone. Other agents are also used.

Barbiturates
The use of barbiturates is reserved for refractory ICP management. Barbiturates and their metabolites take a long time to be eliminated from the body and therefore patients have prolonged periods in ICU following termination of the infusion before they can be assessed neurologically. Hypotension and loss of pupillary constriction complicates barbiturate therapy. Inducing barbiturate coma is often the final therapeutic manoeuvre available for cases with intractable intracranial hypertension and consequently signifies a poorer prognosis.

Surgical management
Mass lesions
All significant mass lesions must be removed as soon as they are diagnosed.
Decompressive craniectomies
Traditionally this has been used as salvage therapy but it is being used more frequently in the aggressive and early management of malignant ICP. The aim is to relieve the constraints of the skull by doing wide craniectomies. Some surgeons do a duraplasty. and leave the dura open. This procedure is associated with a poorer prognosis since the procedure is reserved for patients with refractory raised ICP.

Brain herniation

There may be supratentorial and infratentorial herniation of the brain depending on the nature of the pathology causing the raised intracranial pressure and also the location of that pathology. There are 3 supratentorial herniation syndromes and one infratentorial herniation syndrome:

Subfalcine or cingulate herniation
When the pathology is restricted to a single cerebral hemisphere, the cingulate gyrus may herniate underneath the free edge of the falx cerebri and thus cause midline shift. It is this midline shift that we look for on a trauma CT scan to evaluate whether an extra axial haemorrhage needs to be evacuated. The ventricular system is also displaced and obstructive hydrocephalus may be caused by obstruction of the foramen of Monroe. The anterior cerebral artery or its continuation, the pericallosal artery may be compressed by the edge of the falx cerebri and lead to infarction of the medial cerebral hemispheres.

Uncal herniation (lateral transtentorial herniation)
The uncus is the inferomedial point of the temporal lobe. Masses in the middle fossa cause the temporal lobe to be displaced medially away from the temporal bone. The uncus is compressed against the brainstem and herniates downward into the posterior fossa past the free edge of the tentorium. As the uncus pushes against the brainstem it compresses the ipsilateral oculomotor nerve with resultant ipsilateral pupil dilatation, it also compresses the cerebral peduncle directly and the descending corticospinal tracts (which cross lower down in the medulla) leading to a contralateral hemiparesis.

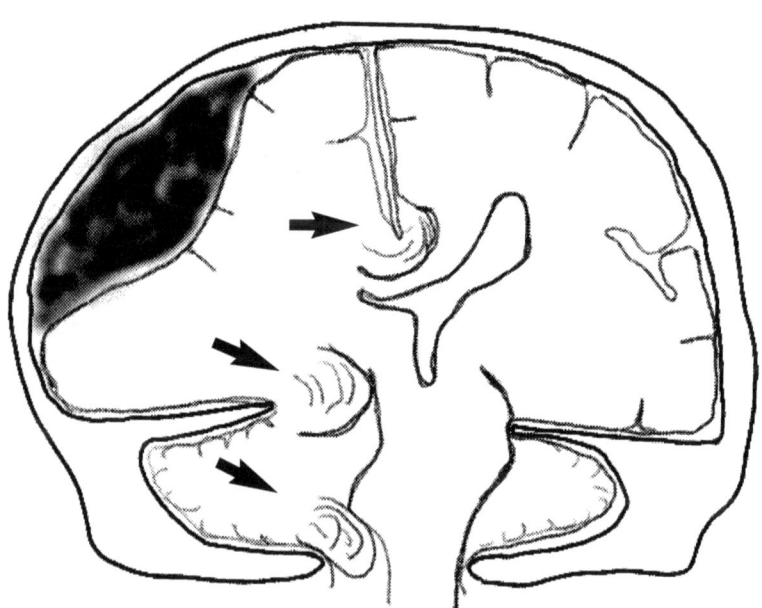

Figure 7. *Brain herniation syndromes. The top arrow demonstrates subfalcine (cingulate) herniation, the middle arrow demonstrates uncal herniation and the last arrow demonstrates tonsillar herniation.*

In Kernohan's paralysis, the brainstem which is being displaced by the uncus is pushed up against the contralateral tentorial edge, causing a notch to form in the brainstem – Kernohan's notch. The contralateral cerebral peduncle is compressed and because the fibres cross lower down, leads to an ipsilateral hemiparesis. The reticular activating system which is located in the brainstem is also compressed leading to impaired consciousness. The posterior cerebral artery may also be compressed at the posterior edge of the tentorial hiatus, causing an occipital lobe infarct.

Central transtentorial herniation
Lesions outside of the middle fossa may cause the diencephalon and midbrain to be pushed through the tentorial hiatus. This leads to patients becoming comatose/obtunded, develop loss of upward gaze, have small reactive pupils and Cheyne-Stokes breathing.

Tonsillar herniation
When there is increased pressure inside the posterior fossa from swelling of the cerebellum or due to a space occupying lesion, the cerebellar tonsils may herniate into the upper spinal canal and thus compress the medulla. This leads to depressed consciousness but also compression of the cardiac and respiratory centres of the midbrain. Hypertension, arrhythmias and abnormal breathing patterns may be seen. Cheyne-Stokes breathing or neurogenic hyperventilation may occur.

Status epilepticus

There are a myriad of causes for epilepsy in a neurosurgical patient. Status epilepticus is associated with severe morbidity and mortality. Status epilepticus can be:

Convulsive status or major motor status is defined as 3 convulsions expressed by major motor twitches with depressed conscious level without patient resurfacing into consciousness, or a single ongoing seizure of more than 30 minutes.
Myoclonic status is when there is a reduced consciousness with myoclonus (shock like contractions of a muscle or muscle group).
Complex partial (temporal lobe seizures with reduced consciousness and automatisms) or absence status is when there is a prolonged period of reduced consciousness that is diagnosed on EEG to be ictal activity.
Subtle status is manifest by minor events such as myoclonic twitches, roving eyes and depressed consciousness.
Epilepsia partialis continuans is focal motor status that does not lead to reduced consciousness.

Overall mortality for status epilepticus is between 10 – 15%. If status persists beyond 4 hours, mortality may be as high as 50% and if it persists beyond 12 hours the mortality is as high as 80%. It is important that all patients with depressed levels of consciousness are intubated to protect their airway. Intravenous access should be established immediately, blood taken for anticonvulsant levels and a 50 ml bolus of 50% dextrose administered. Remember that most anticonvulsants are most effective quite close to or over the toxic level. Epileptic activity should be stopped with a short acting drug and followed by a longer acting drug to control seizures in the longer term (see fig 8).

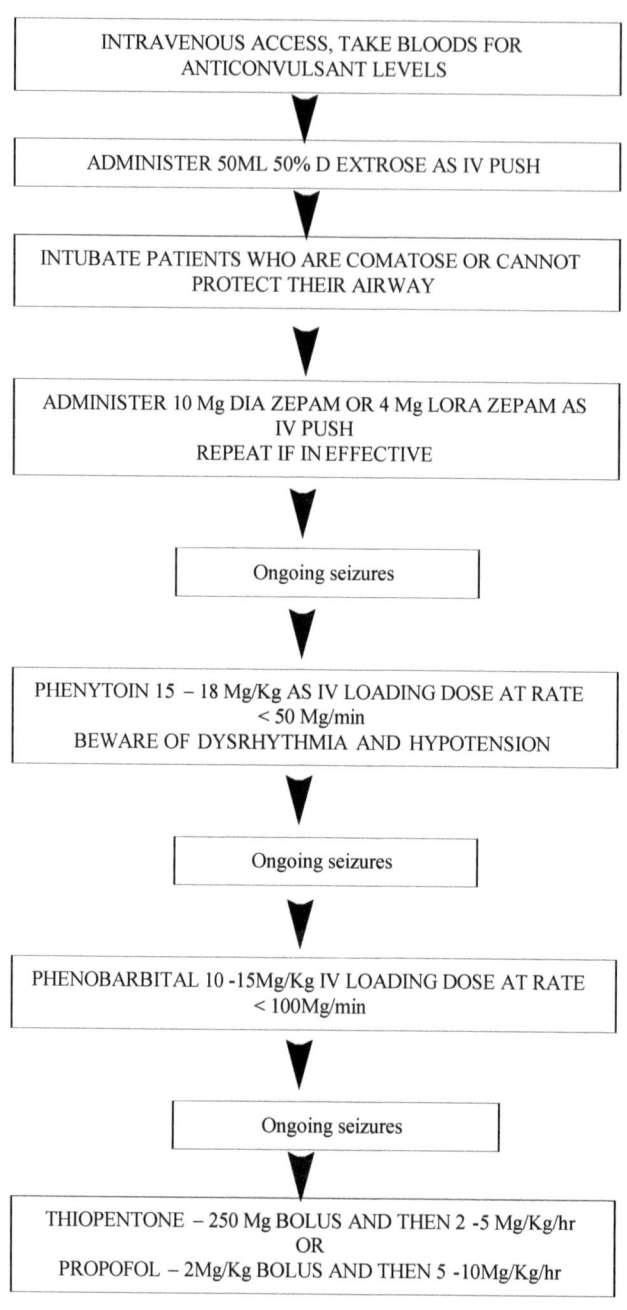

Figure 8. *This flow diagram demonstrates a suggested treatment plan for status epilepticus.*

16

THEATRE

Contents

Introduction
The surgical field
The operating table
Positioning
Skin preparation and draping
Power
Illumination
Instruments
Microscope
Image Guidance
CUSA

Introduction

Operating rooms (OR) depend on the well integrated cooperation of several staff in order to make smooth and efficient running. Before the patient even arrives, the scrub nurse is in charge of preparing and laying out all the appropriate sterile equipment. Sets of instruments vary for each procedure and for each surgeon. When the patient arrives in the anaesthetic room the anaesthetist will put the patient to sleep. Operating department assistants help the anaesthetist and have an important role in the preparation before but also during the operation. Once the operation is under way the scrub nurse is responsible for giving the surgeon all equipment requested in a timely fashion, and it is the verbal and non-verbal communication between an experienced pair of surgeon and scrub nurse that allows the efficient progression of the case. Other than the different roles of the different people in the OR the process also depends on equipment such as the operating table, microscope, surgical tools, intraoperative imaging, and factors such as illumination, ventilation, and the transport of patients to and from the ward.

The surgical field

The patient's position with respect to the floor, the surface of the operating table and the surgeon determine the spatial geometry of the surgical field. Patient positioning is of utmost importance and any time spent positioning the patient appropriately is time well spent; this will save time during the operation itself by ensuring the optimum surgical field is available for operative access and exposure. Positioning of the body and access depends on the different types of operations available.

The operating table

Tables are rigid, flat and heavily structured, to allow secure attachment of other equipment for positioning and to restrain any unwanted patient movement. This also prevents the movement of objects in the operative field. Tables have a segmental structure which is essential in patient positioning; the patient's feet can be placed below the level of the heart to optimise circulation, and the back can be broken in the prone position to flatten the lumbar lordosis in spinal operations. The orientation of the bed itself or parts of it, such as the head, can be rotated, elevated or tilted giving the best surgical field. In procedures where more equipment is needed in the OR, such as image guidance or an image intensifier, the operating table can be moved relative to the doors and equipment to obtain the safest position for surgery. Furthermore, tables are well padded to prevent pressure damage to the patient especially during long procedures. There must be access for the anaesthetist to maintain airway, lines and monitoring. Provision must be available for those cases which might require technical expertise like nerve stimulation, evoked potentials, EMG and EEG.

Positioning

Patient positioning is the art of arranging the body in such a manner so as to give the best surgical access to the surgeon and enhance the surgical field while allowing optimisation of the patient's physiology in terms of CSF drainage, cerebral haemodynamics and cardiorespiratory function. For instance, the torso may be elevated with respect to the extremities to enhance venous drainage, while the head may be raised to 30 degrees to decrease the ICP and the venous pressure in the dural sinuses. As such the surgeon must ensure adequate exposure while maintaining intracranial pressure and haemodynamics. In cranial procedures the chosen position of the head will avoid excessive neck torsion thus reducing venous congestion; account for the effect of posture on cerebral perfusion pressure, cerebral blood flow and CSF flow; and minimise brain retraction by maximising the effect of gravity.

Different positions are customary for different operations. Supine is used for most craniotomies as it allows access to frontal, temporal, parietal and skull base lesions; anterior cervical spine; trans-sphenoidal, trans-oral, petrosal and pterional approaches; and access to the abdomen such as during shunting of CSF. Prone allows access to the posterior parietal and occipital areas of the brain and is used for infratentorial approaches and spinal cases. Care must be taken in such procedures to ensure adequate ventilation; abdominal movement with no compression of the vena cava and subsequent extradural venous haemorrhage; no periorbital trauma; no pressure on genitalia or superficial nerve structures (eg. ulnar nerve, lateral femoral cutaneous nerve of the thigh, common peroneal nerve); and no strain on the axilla and brachial plexus. Special mattresses have been designed for prone procedures, such as the Montreal mattress, although surgeons may prefer an improvised use of pillows and cushioned rolls. The Lateral position provides access for thoracic and lumbar spine operations. It is also used in some cranial cases, whereas it is useful in obese or pregnant patients. Again attention must be paid to structures such as the neck, axilla, appendages and knees. The Sitting position is rather controversial due to cardiopulmonary complications- especially thromboembolism and hypotension- but it may be used for posterior fossa and posterior cervical approaches.

Securing the head in a steady position is achieved with the Mayfield Head Clamp System which employs a three-pin fixation technique on the skull. This ensures that anatomy is maintained after draping. The two-pin end of the clamp is placed on the dependent side of the head, while care is given not to cause a skull fracture by overzealous tightening. The thin squamous temporal bone is therefore avoided and the clamp is placed away from the planned incision site and the eyes.

Skin preparation and draping

Once the patient is positioned by the surgeon and anaesthetist the operative site needs to be prepared. The neurosurgical patient may require head shaving for cranial procedures and the degree of shaving depends on the surgeon. The incision site is marked on the skin in order to maintain anatomical orientation after draping. The skin is then prepared with betadine and/or chlorhexidine antiseptic to provide a sterile field and several layers of surgical drapes/towels are used to cover the patient only leaving exposed the surgical field. A thermal blanket is often used under the draping to maintain normothermia, while a drainage apron may be used for the collection of blood and irrigant solution from the wound.

Power

Whether it is used to power the drills, or supply the heat in diathermy, the modern surgical theatre depends largely on electrical power supply. Gas pressure gradients are also utilised in the suction of fluid from the operative site and for the turning of motorised perforator and craniotome drills; these gradients are achieved by centrally located suction pumps and pressure canisters. Furthermore, the sophisticated OR environment requires a specialised positive ventilation system with respect to surrounding rooms, which is a mechanism against the invasion of infective pathogens.

Illumination

Ambient lighting is supplemented by adjustable Operating Room lighting which uses special reflecting surfaces to focus intense illumination onto the surgical field. Usually these are attached to the ceiling or may be mobile. For a more limited field of view, such as a deep intracerebral tumour cavity, surgeons may also use headlights which provide greater light intensity. Their diasadvantage is that the surgeon remains connected to the light source by a cable running under his/her gown and recquire headgear.

Instruments

The large variety of instruments used in neurosurgery is testament to the several specialised manoeuvres the surgeon is expected to master. To optimise access to instruments during an operation involves the preoperative selection of only those which will be necessary on the surgical field. Others which could be useful but not essential should be on a table nearby. The drapes that form the sterile field also allow the positioning of instruments in such a position so that they are within easy reach of the operative field but do not interfere with the surgeon's economy of movement.

Instruments may be manually controlled or power driven. To perform a burrhole, for example, a manually controlled twist drill can be used or a power drill. The design features of neurosurgical instruments reflect their use and the tissue they are designed to work on. While bone is drilled, perforated, cut and shaped, soft tissue is grasped, divided, separated, retracted, approximated and manipulated. Edges are used in cutting tools like scissors. Teeth, as in forceps, enable a good grasp of tissue; interlocking teeth, as in haemostats or self-retaining retractors, have a 'memory' and remain where placed. Hinge and fulcrum mechanisms allow fine control, such as in bipolar forceps, at a distance and therefore working down a narrow hole.

Haemostasis in neurosurgery is slightly different from other regions as there are usually no big vessel stems to allow the use of ligatures. Bipolar diathermy and the hydrostatic pressure of water in brain cavities are two very important tools.

The surgical field must allow the surgeon enough room for good visualisation and surgical manoeuvre. On one level we have the defining of the surgical field by means of table orientation, patient positioning and draping. While the patient's position on the table will mostly remain stable, the surgeon's view of the surgical field constantly changes. Securing an adequate operative site- especially under a microscope- must be taken to a level higher. Whether it is blood, smoke from cautery or tissue detritus, the surgical site must be kept as clean as possible. This manipulation of the field is achieved by illumination, irrigation and suction.

Specialised instruments have established themselves in neurosurgery: CUSA, Microscope, Image guidance.

Microscope

The introduction of the surgical microscope has revolutionised modern neurosurgery. While the Roman philosopher Pliny referred to magnifying glasses in 1AD, it was a long time before lenses were developed by the Janssen father-and-son team in 16th century Holland. This led to Galileo's first telescope in 1609 and to Anton von Leeuwenhoek and Robert Hooke's experiments in microscopy. The description of the cell by Hooke was only the beginning of a significant medical and scientific advance that was mediated by microscopy. The introduction of microscopes to surgery, nonetheless, did not happen until the 20th century when people like Gazi Yasargil, Jules Hardy and Albert Rhoton helped develop the field of microneurosurgery. The combination of illumination of deep structures and stereoscopic magnification enable the modern neurosurgeon to visualise better, to minimise retractive manoeuvres and perform delicate procedures with the preservation of vital or eloquent structures.

The microscope components include adjustable eyepieces; a binocular tube with rotational ability for comfort and adjustability of the interpupillary distance for depth perception; a lens-based magnification adjuster system (zoom and focus); a control panel for zoom and focus changes as well as repositioning capability; and a base with light source. The microscope is set up and prepared before the operation both for the surgeon and the assistant, whose position may be adjusted to the side or opposite to the surgeon. Microscopes are draped in a sterile fashion and space should be allowed in the OR for their moving into close range of the surgical field. Intraoperative changes of the position of the microscope are necessary to view all corners of the surgical field and indirect hand-eye coordination is a skill acquired through practice. To enhance dexterity armrest or forearm support in the seated position is used in cranial work whereas commonly the microscope is used in the standing position for spinal surgery.

Image Guidance

The integration of the operating microscope into a frameless stereotactical navigational system is an exciting tool in neurosurgery. Microscopic angle and focal length are digitalised and incorporated into an infrared localising system. Such information is compared to data from CT or MRI that have been entered into the guidance system, to create a 3-dimensional reconstruction of anatomical pathology that guides the surgeon in relation to normal anatomy and surgical equipment. The advantages include more precision in approach, limited surgical exposure, greater safety and more complete tumour removal. Skin markers are registered using a probe which is linked to the computer by a camera which detects the probe's position in space. This marries the position of the head in space with the images in the computer. Surgical instruments incorporating light emitting diodes are followed by the computer during the operation. The surgeon can navigate through the brain using the computer images linked to his surgical instruments or microscope.

CUSA

The CUSA® (cavitational ultrasonic surgical aspirator) generates forces that fragment the cells. It consists of a hollow titanium tip that vibrates on its longitudinal axis and mechanical energy is transferred when the tip of the instrument is brought in contact with tissue, thus creating low and high pressure areas. When the pressure is below the vapour pressure of tissue fluid, vapour-filled vacuoles form within the cells, which vacuoles then expand or collapse as pressure rises or falls with each cycle. Tissue damage is confined to an area of about 25 to 50μm next to the tip, with minimal thermal injury and protein denaturation, a much lesser damage than from a scalpel, laser, or electrosurgery. Another advantage of CUSA® system is selectivity of dissection and depends on the water content of cells; different tissues fragment at different rates, and dissection may leave blood vessels and connective tissue skeletonised and intact.

17

FURTHER READING

Contents

Journals: Basic science
Journals: Clinical
Texts: Basic science
Texts: Clinical

Please find below a selection of excellent texts.

Journals: Basic science
Science
Nature
Nature Neuroscience
Nature Reviews in Neuroscience
Neuron
Cell
Trends in Neurological Sciences
Journal of Neuroscience
Neuroscience
Journal of Physiology
American Journal of Physiology
Proceedings of the National Academy of Science
Journal of Neurobiology
Journal of Comparative Neurology
Brain
Cerebral Cortex
Synapse

Journals: Clinical
Lancet
Lancet Neurology
New England of Medicine
British Medical Journal
Cochrane Reviews
Neurosurgery Clinics of North America
Journal of Neurosurgery
Neurosurgery

Acta Neurochirurgica
British Journal of Neurosurgery
Surgical Neurology
Neurosurgical Focus
Neurosurgery Quarterly
Clinical Neurology and Neurosurgery
Journal of Neurology Neurosurgery and Psychiatry
Journal of Neurosurgery: Pediatrics
Child's Nervous System
Pediatric Neurosurgery
Journal of Neurosurgery: Spine
Spine
European Spine
Journal of Bone and Joint Surgery
Minimally Invasive Neurosurgery
Strereotactic and Functional Neurosurgery
Movement Disorders
Journal of Neurooncology
Acta Neuropathologica
Neuroradiology

Texts: Basic science
Neuroanatomy
The Whole Brain Atlas at www.med.harvard.edu/AANLIB/home.html
Kandel ER, Schwartz JH, Jessell TM. Principles of Neural Science, 4th edition, McGraw-Hill/Appleton & Lange, 2000.
Martin JH. Neuroanatomy: Text and Atlas, McGraw-Hill/Appleton & Lange, 2003.
Haines DE. Neuroanatomy: An Atlas of Structures, Sections, and Systems, 5th edition, Lippincott Williams & Wilkins, 2002.
Hendelman WJ. Atlas of Functional Neuroanatomy, CRC Press, 2000.

Neurophysiology
Kandel ER, Schwartz JH, Jessell TM. Principles of Neural Science, 4th edition, McGraw-Hill/Appleton & Lange, 2000.
Carpenter RHS. Neurophysiology, 4th edition, Arnold Publishers, 2002.

Neuropathology
Greenfield JG, Lantos PL and Graham DI. Greenfield's Neuropathology (2 Volumes), 7th edition, Arnold Publishers, 2002.
Nelson JS. Principles and Practice of Neuropathology, 2nd edition, Oxford University Press, 2003.

Microbiology of the CNS
Osenbach RK and Zeidman SM. Infections in Neurological Surgery: Diagnosis and Management, Lippincott Williams & Wilkins, 1998.
Hall WA and McCutcheon IC. Infections in Neurosurgery, Thieme Medical Publishers, 2000.

Texts: Clinical

History of neurosurgery
Greenblatt SH, Dagi TF and Epstein MH (eds). A History of Neurosurgery. In its scientific and Professional Contexts, The American Association of Neurological Surgeons, 1997.

General neurology
Patten JP. Neurological Differential Diagnosis, 2nd edition, Springer, 1998.
Greenberg D, Aminoff MJ and Simon RP. Clinical Neurology, 5th edition, McGraw-Hill/Appleton & Lange, 2002.
Jones Jr HR and Netter FH. Netter's Neurology, Novartis Medical Education, 2004.

General neurosurgery
Introductory texts:
Black PMcL and Rossitch E. Neurosurgery: An Introductory Text, Oxford University Press, 1995.
Lindsay KW and Bone I. Neurology and Neurosurgery Illustrated, 4th edition, Churchill Livingstone, 2004.
Kaye AH. Essential Neurosurgery, 3rd edition, Blackwell Publishers, 2005.
Liebenberg WA, Neurosurgery for Non Neurosurgeons, Vesuvius Books, 2006.
Liebenberg WA and Johnson RD. Neurosurgery for Basic Surgical Trainees, Hippocrates Books, 2004.
Liebenberg WA. Neurosurgery Explained, Vesuvius Books, 2006

Specialised texts:
Greenberg MS. Handbook of Neurosurgery, 5th edition, Berlin: Thieme Publishers, 2001.
Winn RH (ed). Youman's Neurological Surgery, 5th edition, W. B Saunders, 2004.
Rengachary SS and Ellenbogen RG. Principles of Neurosurgery, 2nd edition, Mosby, 2004.
Awad I. Philosophy of Neurological Surgery, Thieme/AANS, 1995.

Operative Surgery
Rhoton Jr AL. Cranial anatomy and surgical approaches. Lippincott William & Wilkins/CNS, 2003.
Kaye AH and Black PMcL. Operative Neurosurgery, Churchill Livingstone, 2000.
Schmidek HH and Sweet WH. Schmidek & Sweet's Operative Neurosurgical Techniques: Indications, Methods, and Results, 4th edition, Elsevier, 2000.
Conolly ES, McKhann GM, Huang J and Choudhri TF. Fundamentals of Operative Techniques in Neurosurgery, Thieme Medical Publishers, 2002.
Day JD, Koos WT, Matula C and Lang J. Color Atlas of Microneurosurgical Approaches, Thieme Medical Publishers, 1997.
Fossett DT and Caputy AJ. Operative Neurosurgical Anatomy, Thieme Medical Publishers, 2002.
Sekhar L and de Oliveira E. Cranial Microsurgery: Approaches and Technique. Thieme Medical Publishers, 1999.
Yasargil MG. Microneurosurgery (Volumes 1-4), Thieme Medical Publishers, 1984-1996.

Trauma
Valadka AB and Andrews BT. Neurotrauma: Evidence-Based Answers to Common

Questions. Thieme Medical Publishers, 2005.
Marion D. Traumatic Brain Injury. Thieme Medical Publishers, 1999.

Neuro-critical care
Andrews BT (ed). Intensive Care in Neurosurgery, Thieme, 2003.
Suarez JI (ed). Critical Care Neurology and Neurosurgery, Humana Press, 2004.

Neuroradiology/ Interventional neuroradiology
Osborn AG and Maak J. Diagnostic Neuroradiology, Mosby, 1994.
Kirkwood JR. Essentials of Neuroimaging, 2nd edition, Churchill Livingstone, 1995.
Byrne JV (ed). Interventional Neuroradiology: Theory and Practice, Oxford University Press, 2002.
Osborn A, Blaser S and Salzman K. Diagnostic Imaging: Brain, W.B. Saunders, 2004.
Hosten N and Liebig T (translated by Telger TC). CT of the Head and Spine, Thieme Medical Publishers, 2002.

Neurovascular
Byrne JV (ed). Interventional Neuroradiology: Theory and Practice, Oxford University Press, 2002.
Grand W and Hopkins LN. Vasculature of the Brain and Cranial Base. Thieme Medical Publishers, 1999.
Ojemann RG and Ogilvy CS. Surgical Management of Neurovascular Disease, 3rd edition, Williams & Wilkins, 1995.

Neuro-oncology
Berger MS and Prados M. Textbook of Neuro-Oncology, Elsevier/Saunders, 2004.
Apuzzo MJ. Benign Cerebral Gliomas, Volumes I and II, 1995, Thieme/AANS.
Fischer G and Brotchi J. Intramedullary Spinal Cord Tumors, Thieme Medical Publishers, 1996.

Skull Base
Dolenc VV and Rogers L. Microsurgical Anatomy and Surgery of the Central Skull Base, Springer, 2003.
Sen C, Chen CS and Post KD. Microsurgical Anatomy of the Skull Base and Approaches to the Cavernous Sinus. Thieme Medical Publishers, 1997.

Spine
Benzel EC. Spine Surgery, Churchill Livingstone, 2004.
Haher TR and Merola AA Surgical Techniques of the Spine, Thieme Medical Publishers, 2003.
Devlin VJ. Spine Secrets, Hanley & Belfus, 2003.
Vaccaro A, Betz RR and Zeidman. SM Principles and Practice of Spine Surgery, Mosby, 2002.
Benzel E. Biomechanics of Spine Stabilisation, Thieme/AANS, 2001.

Peripheral nerves
Maniker A. Operative Exposures In Peripheral Nerve Surgery, Thieme Medical Publishers, 2004.
Kline DG. Atlas of Peripheral Nerve Surgery, 2nd edition, W.B. Saunders, 2001.

Functional neurosurgery
Schulder M. Handbook of Stereotactic and Functional Neurosurgery, Marcel Dekker Ltd, 2003.
Gildenberg PL and Tasker RR. Textbook of Stereotactic and Functional Neurosurgery, McGraw-Hill, 1997.
Germano I. Neurosurgical Treatment of Movement Disorders, Thieme/AANS, 1998.

Pain
Burchiel K. Surgical Management of Pain, Thieme Medical Publishers, 2002.

Neuroendocrinology
Powell MP, Lightman SL and Laws Jr ER. Management of Pituitary Tumors: The Clinician's Practical Guide, 2nd edition, Humana Press, 2003.

Pediatric neurosurgery
Choux M, Hockley AD and Di Rocco C. Pediatric Neurosurgery, Churchill Livingstone, 1999.
McLaurin RL and McLone D. Pediatric Neurosurgery: Surgery of the Developing Nervous System, Saunders, 2000.
Albright AL, Pollack IF and Adelson PD (eds). Operative Techniques in Pediatric Neurosurgery, Thieme Medical Publishers, 2000.

A

abbreviated mental test score 15, 17
Abscess 32, 50, 68, 69, 141
acceleration–deceleration 42
acoustic neuroma 100
ADH 172
ambient 38
ambient cistern 38
Anaplastic astrocytoma 31, 49, 50
aneurysm 110, 111, 112, 114, 115
aneurysms 109, 110, 111, 113, 114, 115
angiography 110, 113, 114
Angiomas 140
annulus 142, 143, 145
annulus fibrosus 142, 143, 145
anterior longitudinal ligament 132, 133
anterior vertebral line 73, 75
aqueduct 35
aqueduct of Sylvius 35, 122, 123
Arachnoid cyst 31, 55, 56, 71, 87
arachnoid granulations 156
Arterial infarct 32, 62
Arteriovenous Malformation 32, 66, 67, 72, 91
Arteriovenous malformations 109
Astrocytes 95
astrocytoma 31, 32, 48, 49, 50, 60, 71, 85, 95, 104, 105
astrocytomas 140
ataxia 100
atherosclerotic plaques 109
atlanto – occipital dissociation 74
atlanto-dens interval 74, 75
AVM 109, 110, 115
AVMs 111, 115
Axonotmesis 148

B

Babinski 28
Barbiturates 173

basal cisterns 37, 38, 40, 44, 45, 47, 55, 63, 65, 66
bilirubin 45, 113
BIS 161, 167, 168, 169
Bispectral analysis 161, 167
bitemporal hemianopia 18, 99
Bony tumours 71, 78, 101
brain cell ischaemia 170
Brain herniation 161, 174
Brain injury 128
Brain oedema 33, 62
Brain tissue oxygen tension monitoring 161, 167
brain tumour 97
brain tumours 31, 34, 48, 95, 96, 97, 98
Broca's area 28

C

Carpal tunnel syndrome 149
cartilage producing tumours 71, 78
Cartilaginous tumours 102
cauda equina 76, 78, 90
cavernoma 92
cavernomas 109, 110
Cavernous angioma 72, 92
Cavernous angiomas 109, 110
Cavernous malformation 32, 67, 92
cavernous malformations 109
Cavernous sinus 99
cavitational ultrasonic surgical aspirator 181
CBV 124
Central neurocytomas 31, 57
Central transtentorial herniation 175
Cerebellopontine angle 98, 100, 123
Cerebellum 100, 105
Cerebral aneurysms 109, 110
cerebral arterial oxygenation 165
cerebral ischaemia 118, 119
cerebral oedema 42, 121, 122
cerebral perfusion pressure 113
cerebral salt wasting 172
Cerebritis 32, 68

cerebrospinal fluid 121
Cervical spine 126, 129, 130, 133, 135, 136, 141, 142, 143, 144, 145
cervical spondylosis 77, 139, 142, 143
Chemotherapy 98, 102, 103, 104
cholesteotoma 100
Chondrosarcoma 102, 106, 107
chorda tympani 22
Chordoma 32, 60, 71, 81, 103, 107
Choroid plexus 95, 105
Choroid plexus papilloma 95, 105
cingulate herniation 174
circle of Willis 110, 111, 118
clivus 99
cochlear nerve 22
Colloid cyst 31, 40, 42, 54, 55, 123
Comminuted fractures 127
communicating hydrocephalus 40, 41, 65, 112, 156
Congenital abnormalities 151
conus 83
Convulsive status 175
coronal suture 39
CPP 113, 161, 162, 166, 169, 170, 171, 173
cranial nerve palsy 97, 100
Cranial nerves 15, 20, 22, 24, 126, 128
craniopharyngioma 96, 106
Craniopharyngiomas 31, 57
craniovertebral junction 136
CSF 33, 34, 37, 38, 41, 42, 45, 54, 55, 56, 60, 68, 96, 99, 112, 113, 121, 122, 123, 151, 153
CSW 172
CT 31, 32, 33, 35, 36, 38, 39, 40, 41, 42, 43, 44, 45, 46, 47, 48, 49, 50, 51, 52, 53, 54, 55, 56, 57, 58, 59, 60, 61, 62, 63, 64, 65, 66, 67, 68, 69
Cubital tunnel syndrome 149
CUSA 177, 180, 181
CVP 114
Cytotoxic oedema 122

DBI 42
Decompressive craniectomies 173

Demyelination 34
deoxyhaemoglobin 45
Depressed fractures 127, 131
dermatome 24, 28
Dermoid cyst 31, 54, 71, 87, 89
Dermoid cysts 96, 104
Dermoid tumours 33
Developmental abnormalities 151, 153
Diffuse Brain Injury 31, 42, 44, 45
diplopia 19, 20, 100
Disc herniation 71, 74
disc prolapse 75, 76, 78
disc protrusion 140, 143, 144, 145, 146
Discitis 72, 89, 90, 93
dorsum sellae 43, 99
Dural arteriovenous fistula 72, 91
dynamic perfusion CT 114
dysdiadocokinesia 25

Endocrine disturbances 96
echo time 34
ectoderm 151, 152
Edinger Westphal 20
Edinger-Westphal 20, 21
EEG 161, 167, 169, 175
Ehlers-Danlos syndrome 110
elastance curve 170, 171
Empbryonic 95
Empyema 32, 68
endovascular embolisaton 115
endovascular treatment 114, 115
Entrapment neuropathies 147, 149
ependyma 85, 95
Ependymoma 31, 51, 71, 83, 85, 95, 104, 105
ependymomas 85, 140
Epidermoid cyst 31, 54, 71, 87, 100
epidermoid cysts 104
Epidural abscess 156, 157, 158, 159
epidural abscesses 140

Epidural empyema 72, 90
Epidural haematoma 72, 93
Epilepsy 96, 97, 99, 112
ethmoid sinuses 96
Evoked potentials 169
Ewing sarcoma 103
Extension 133, 134
Extra axial 31
Extradural 95, 101, 103
Eye opening response 28, 30

F

facial nerve 22
False aneurysms 110
falx 37, 38, 41, 52
falx cerebri 41
Filum terminale ependymomas 104
Fisher grading scale 64
FLAIR 33, 34, 50, 53, 54, 55
flexion rotation injuries 133
flow voids 91
fluid attenuation inversion recovery 33, 34
Focal neurological deficits 96, 97
focal neurological deficits 128
foramen of Luschka 100
fourth ventricle 35, 38, 40, 41, 51, 65, 66, 122, 123, 157
frontal lobe 43, 44
fundoscopy 18, 19, 24

G

Gait 26, 27, 97
Gamma knife 12
Gangliocytoma 95, 105
ganglioglioma 95, 105
Gangliogliomas 104
Germinoma 32, 58
Glasgow Coma Scale 28
Glial tumours 33, 60
Glioblastoma 31, 49, 50, 95, 104, 105

Glioblastoma Multiforme 31, 50
glossopharyngeal nerve 23
gradient echo 33

Haemangioblastoma 71, 86, 96
Haematomas 141
HAEMORRHAGE 117, 118
head injuries 125, 127, 129, 130
head injury 125, 126, 128, 129, 130
Hemangioblastoma 32, 59
Herring-Traube-Mayer waves 163
HHH therapy 114, 115
homonomous hemianopia 18
Homonymous hemianopia 99
Horner's syndrome 21
Hounsfield 33, 46
hydrocephalus 31, 35, 40, 41, 42, 51, 54, 55, 57, 58, 59, 63, 65, 96, 99, 100, 101, 112, 115, 121, 122, 123, 151, 153, 156, 157, 158
hydromyelia 28
hydrostatic pressure 41
Hypernatremia 172
Hypertension 109, 111, 112
hypertensive haemorrhage 32, 66
hyperventilation 171, 175
Hyponatremia 172
hypothalamus 96

ICH 112, 113, 117, 118
ICP 96, 97, 98, 99, 100, 101, 117, 118, 119, 161, 162, 163, 164, 169, 170, 171, 172, 173
Image Guidance 177, 178, 180, 181
induced hypothermia 171
infarction 109, 112, 113, 114, 115, 117, 118, 119
intervertebral 132, 133
intervertebral disc 72, 73, 74, 76, 78, 90, 132
intervertebral joints 143, 145
Intracerebral abscess 157, 158

intra-cerebral haematoma 96, 97, 112
Intracerebral haemorrhage 31, 44, 66
Intracranial compliance 163, 170
Intracranial elastance 170
Intracranial infections 155
Intracranial pressure monitoring 161, 162, 163
intracranial volume 170
Intradural, extramedullary 95, 101, 103
intramedullary 71, 79, 85, 87, 91, 92, 95, 101, 104
Intramedullary abscess 159
inversion recovery 33, 34
isodense 33, 47, 50, 51, 54, 56

J

Jugular Venous Oximetry 165
JVO 165, 166

K

Kernig's sign 112

L

lambdoid 39
lateral geniculate body 18, 20
lateral rectus 19
lateral ventricle 37, 41, 42, 65, 69
lateral ventricles 35, 37, 40, 42, 64, 65
ligamentum flavum 74, 76, 77, 142, 143, 144, 145
limb weakness 97
Linear fractures 127
Linnac particle beam accelerator 12
lipomas 104, 140
LP 121
lumbar puncture 121
Lumbar spondylosis 139, 142, 145
Lundberg 163, 164
Lundberg's A 121
Luschka 122
lymphoma 31, 53, 71, 79, 96, 102

Lymphoproliferative tumours 71, 79, 102

M

Macroadenomas 31, 56
Magnetic Resonance Imaging 33
major motor status 175
MAP 170, 171, 172, 173
Marcus Gunn pupil 21
Marfan syndrome 110
Marshall classification 44
Mayo Clinic scale 25
Measurement of cerebral blood flow 161, 165
medulla oblongata 24
Medulloblastoma 32, 59, 95, 106
melanoma 95, 107
Meninges 95, 96, 106, 126, 128
Meningioma 31, 52, 53, 71, 82, 95, 106, 140
meningiomas 84, 97, 98, 99, 100, 103, 140
Meningitis 155, 156, 157, 158
meningocoele 153
meningo-myelocoele 153
Meralgia paraesthetica 150
Metastatic 32, 34, 61
Metastatic tumours 71, 81, 95, 96, 103, 107
Meyer's loop 18
Microadenomas 31, 56
Microdialysis 167
microdiscectomy 146
Microscope 177, 180, 181
mini mental state examination 15
Mini Mental Status Examination 16
Monroe – Kelly doctrine 169
Morton's syndrome 150
Motor dysfunction 137
Motor evoked potentials 169
Motor response 28, 30
motor system 24, 26, 27
motor weakness 27
Moya Moya disease 111
MRC Scale 25

MRI 31, 32, 33, 34, 35, 38, 39
Multiple myeloma 71, 79, 80, 102
mural nodule 86
mycobacterium tuberculosis 90
myelocoele 153
Myxopapillary ependymoma 71, 83

N

Near infrared spectroscopy 166
neo-vascularity 48
NERVE ENTRAPMENT 147
Nerve sheath tumours 103
Neural crest 151, 152
Neural fold 152
Neural foramina 72, 73, 83
Neural groove 151, 152
Neural plate 152
Neurenteric cyst 72, 87
Neurilemmoma 95
neuroblastoma 95, 105, 106
neuroectoderm 151
Neuroepithelial 95, 96, 105
neurofibroma 83, 84, 95, 107, 140
Neurofibromas 103, 140
neurofibromatosis type 1 110
Neurological examination 14, 15
Neuromuscular blockade 173
Neuronal tumours 31, 57
Neuropraxia 148
Neurotmesis 148
NIRS 166
non-communicating 40
nystagmus 100

O

Obstructive hydrocephalus 40, 42, 54, 55
occipital cortex 15
Occipital neuralgia 150
odontoid peg 74

oedema 170, 173
Oligodendrocytes 95
Oligodendroglioma 31, 51, 95, 105
Operating rooms 177
operating table 177, 178
optic chiasm 20, 99
Optic nerve 99
optic radiation 18
Optic tract 99
Osteoblastoma 71, 79, 101
Osteochondroma 71, 79, 102
Osteoid osteoma 71, 78, 79, 101
Osteomyelitis 72, 89, 90, 93
osteophytes 143, 145
Osteosarcoma 101, 102

PaCO2 124
pain fibres 28
papilloedema 19, 21, 161
Paraganglioma 71, 84, 86
Paramagnetic 33, 34
Patient positioning 177, 178, 180
PAWP 114
pedicle 73, 81, 83, 85, 86
penetrating injuries 133, 134
perfusion imaging 114
Perineural cyst 71, 87
peripheral nerves 147, 150
photophobia 112
Physical Examination 14
Pilocytic astrocytoma 31, 50
Pineal gland 95, 98
Pineal parenchymal tumours 32, 58
Pinealoblastoma 59
Pinealocytoma 58
Pineoblastoma 95, 105, 106
Pineocytoma 95, 105, 106
Pituitary 9, 96, 97, 98, 99, 100, 106
polycystic kidney disease 110

Pons 100, 101
posterior commisure 20
posterior inferior cerebellar arteries 100
posterior longitudinal ligament 74
posterior vertebral line 73, 75
prepontine 38
Primary brain tumours 95, 96
Primitive neuro-ectodermal tumour 59
proprioception 24, 25, 27, 28
Proton density 34
pulse sequences 33

Q

quadrigeminal 38
quadrigeminal cistern 38
Queckenstedt's test 121

R

radiculopathy 24, 143, 144, 145
Radiotherapy 98, 100, 102, 103
Raised ICP 112, 113, 121, 122, 124, 129, 156, 157, 161, 162, 170, 173
raised intracranial pressure 96, 121, 161, 169, 174
raised intra-cranial pressure 118, 121
reflexes 24, 26, 27, 28
repetition time 33
retina 15, 18, 20
Rheumatoid arthritis 71, 74
rhizotomies 10
Rinne's test 23
Round cell tumours 103

S

sagittal sinus 63
SAH 63, 64, 65, 109, 111, 112, 113, 114, 115
Scalp injuries 126
Schwannoma 71, 83
schwannomas 103
Schwanomas 100

Secondary brain damage 125, 129
Seddon's classification 148
seizures 109, 113
Sensory dysfunction 137
Sensory evoked potentials 169
septum pellucidum 41
short tau inversion recovery 34
SIADH 172
Signal Quality Index 169
single photon emission computed tomography 114
Skull 126, 127, 128, 131
Skull base 9
Skull fractures 31, 42
Snellen chart 15
SOL 161, 162
Solitary plasmacytoma 71, 79, 102
space occupying lesion 122, 161, 175
space occupying lesions 96, 97
SPECT 114
spectroscopy 113
speech 97
Spetzler-Martin grading scale 109, 110
Sphenoid sinus 99, 100
sphenoid sinuses 96
spina bifida occulta 151, 153
Spinal 9
spinal accessory nerve 23
Spinal canal stenosis 143, 146
spinal cord 72, 73, 74, 77, 82, 83, 92, 93
Spinal cord compression 139, 140, 141, 142, 143, 144
Spinal Infections 155, 158
spinal injuries 125, 136
spinal injury 125, 132, 133, 134, 136
Spinal stenosis 71, 74, 76
Spinal tumours 71, 78, 95, 101
spinolaminar line 73, 75
spontaneous haemorrhage 109
Spontaneous haemorrhages 109
Status epilepticus 161, 175, 176
Stereotactic irradiation 98
sternomastoid 101

STIR 34, 54
subarachnoid 32, 33, 38, 40, 44, 63, 65
Subarachnoid haemorrhage 32, 44
subarachnoid heamorrhage 109, 111
subdural 42, 43, 45, 46, 47, 68
Subdural abscess 157, 159
subdural empyema 157
subdural haematoma 43, 45, 46, 47, 72, 92
subdural haemorrhage 42, 45
Sunderland classification 148
superior colliculus 20
superior oblique 19, 20
Suppression Ratio 169
supra sellar region 100
supra sellar tumours 99
supratentorial herniation 174
syndrome of inappropriate ADH 172
Synovial cyst 72, 87, 88
syringomyelia 28, 86

T

Tarlov cyst 71, 87
Tarsal tunnel syndrome 150
TCD 165
temporal bone 41, 43, 46
temporal horn 41, 65
temporal visual field 18
Thalamic 123
The surgical field 177, 178, 179, 180
third ventricle 31, 35, 38, 40, 41, 42, 54, 55, 58, 63, 65
Tinnitus 101
Tissue intensities 31, 34
Tonsillar herniation 161, 162, 174, 175
Transcranial Doppler Ultrasonography 165
transmembrane pumps 170
trapezius 101
Trigeminal 22
Trigeminal neuralgia 150
trigone 37, 41
Tuberculosis 72, 90

Tumours of notochordal origin 103

U

Uncal herniation 174
uncus 46
upper quadrant hemianopia 18
upper quadrantanopia 18

V

vagus 23
Vascular anomalies 32, 66
Vasculitis 111
Vasogenic oedema 122, 157
vasopressin 172
Vasospasm 111, 112, 113, 114, 115
Venous angioma 32, 67
Venous infarct 32, 63
Ventriculostomy 123, 173
Verbal response 28, 30
vertebrae 132
Vertical compression 133
vertigo 100, 101, 128
vestibular nerve 22
Vestibular schwannoma 32, 38, 60, 100
Visual acuity 15, 18
visual confrontation testing 18, 19
Visual field 99
Visual fields 15, 18, 19

W

Wallerian degeneration 148
Weber's test 23
WFNS 113, 115
WFNS grade 113
WHO classification 95, 105
World Federation of Neurological Surgeons 113

X

Xenon CT 114

www.ingramcontent.com/pod-product-compliance
Ingram Content Group UK Ltd.
Pitfield, Milton Keynes, MK11 3LW, UK
UKHW021319180426
11947UKWH00015B/1329